AF872199

THE ULTIMATE GP TRAINING APPLICATION GUIDE

UniAdmissions

ISBN: 978-1-915091-20-8

Published by RAR Medical Services Limited
www.uniadmissions.co.uk
info@uniadmissions.co.uk
Tel: +44 (0) 208 068 0438

ABOUT THE AUTHOR

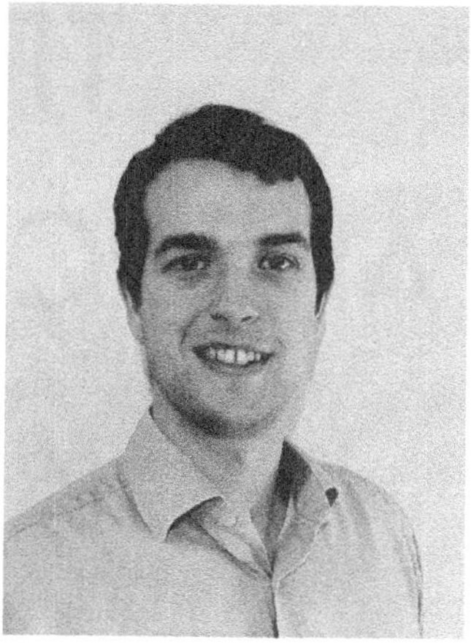

Simon is a member of The Royal College of General Practitioners and completed his General Practice Specialty training in Nottingham. He currently works as a GP in a city centre training practice. He has an interest in health inequalities and is currently developing expertise in public health research alongside working as a GP.

Outside of work Simon enjoys long-distance running and is an avid watcher of cricket.

THE ULTIMATE GP TRAINING APPLICATION GUIDE

DR SIMON BAILEY

UniAdmissions

CONTENTS

PREFACE

There is tremendous privilege in being a General Practitioner. By working in Primary care, GPs help to provide the 'front door' of the NHS and can advocate for our patients to the wider healthcare system. GPs are allowed a continuity of care that can span decades and generations and can develop a professional intimacy with patients that is difficult to match in other specialties. As a vital service to the community patients will come to see you in their time of need but will also be quick to tell you any good news too. You will be allowed into people's homes and to care for their most loved ones.

Although GPs are generalists by name, a GP becomes a master in consultation skills, listening and history taking. A GP needs to problem solve and deal with medical complexity. They do not know what will come through the door next and need to be prepared whether it be mundane or an emergency. The ability to empathise and act holistically allows a GP to tailor their care to the patient and build a trust between the patient and not just the Doctor but the health service itself.

The role of the GP is evolving. More care is being moved into the community and the population is growing. This has raised pressures as well as caused remodelling to services. The multi-disciplinary team that now operates requires the leadership and management of general practice and there is much to the role beyond the consulting room. The use of technology is helping GPs to work efficiently and effectively despite challenging conditions. There is also a lot of opportunity to develop a portfolio career or to develop a flexible work pattern to aid other responsibilities and this trend is likely to continue into the future.

When applying for the General Practice Training programme it is not expected that you are the finished article. However, through understanding the role and attributes required to be a GP you will maximise the potential of your application and time during training.

THE BASICS

THE GP TRAINING PROGRAMME

GP specialty training is usually a 3 year programme starting at ST1. During these 3 years there will be a mix of posts in general practice and in hospital. The posts are either 4 or 6 months and at least 18 months in total will be spent in general practice. Some deaneries offer longer time in General Practice.

The hospital posts will vary between trainees. Specialties include but are not limited to Emergency Medicine, ENT, Obstetrics and gynaecology, paediatrics, general medicine, dermatology and psychiatry. There may be some allowance made for doctors who already have experience in a specialty e.g. in foundation years or other specialty training but this is not guaranteed. It should be understood that you are a GP trainee during these posts and thus the role and responsibilities may differ from a specialty trainee of the same grade. An example of this would be that an obstetric and gynaecology ST2 may be expected to take a more active role in theatre or responsibility on the labour ward than a GPST2 doing a short post.

The last 12 months of training (ST3) should be in a general practice post and you should be working in the same practice for this time. This gives valuable experience in the specialty and for many is the first time in a career that they have not had to change posting after a few months.

Example programme:

- Emergency Medicine – hospital post 4 months
- General practice – 4 months
- Geriatric medicine – 4 months
- Obstetric and gynaecology – 4 months
- General practice – 4 months
- Psychiatry – 4 months
- General practice – 12 months

This is an example of a GP training programme however there is likely to be variability in the length of posts and the variety of posts depending on the deanery and local services. This programme does not have a paediatrics post and therefore the trainee would miss out on this experience. They would be expected to demonstrate the relevant competencies regarding paediatrics to complete their training and would likely need to focus more on this during their general practice posts.

Applying for the programme

General Practice ST1 recruitment is managed through the GP National Recruitment Office (GPNRO) and applications take place through the Oriel online portal. Suitable applicants will be allowed to register for the Multi-Specialty Recruitment Assessment.

The MSRA is a computer-based test and a mix of professional dilemma and clinical problem solving questions. This is the most important part of the application process as the results determine your applicant ranking. The MSRA will be covered in depth later in this book.

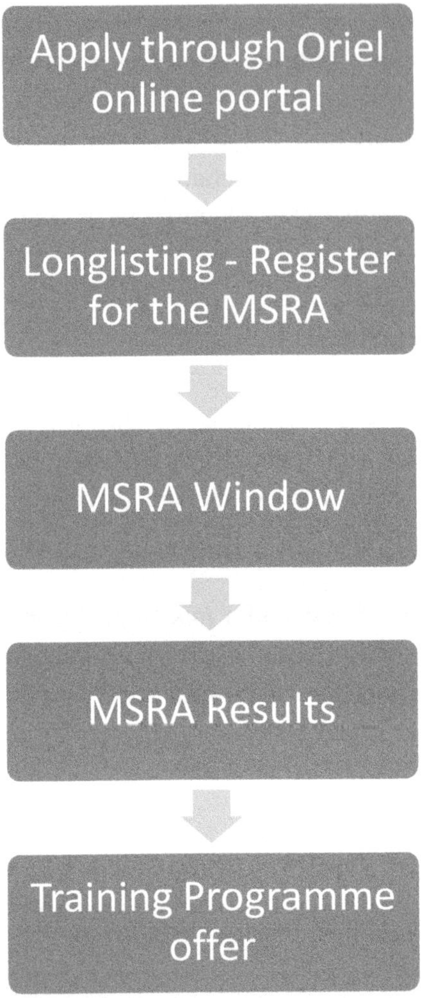

ELIGIBILITY

Health Education England produce a Person Specification for recruitment to GP specialty training. In order to be eligible applicants must:

- Be eligible for full registration with, and hold a current licence to practise from the GMC at intended start date

- Have evidence of achievement of foundation competences, in the three and a half years preceding the advertised post start date for the round of application, via one of the following methods:
  - Current employment in a UKFPO-affiliated foundation programme (this means that you are a current FY2 doctor) ; **or**
  - Having been awarded an FPCC (Foundation Programme Certificate of Completion) from a UK affiliated foundation programme within the 3.5 years preceding the advertised post start date (you have completed your Foundation training in the last 3.5 years) ; **or**
  - Current employment in a GMC approved Specialty Training Programme holding either a National Training Number (NTN) or Deanery Reference Number (DRN) (you are currently a trainee on a different programme looking to change to GP); **or**
  - 12 months medical experience after full GMC registration (or equivalent post licensing experience), and evidence to commence specialty training in the form of a *Certificate of Readiness to Enter Specialty Training*
- Be eligible to work in the UK
- Eligible for UK Medical Performers' Lists (This is a list of doctors working in primary care)
- Hold a current and in date valid driving licence or provides an undertaking to provide alternative means of transport when providing emergency and domiciliary care to fulfil the requirements of the whole training programme

The GP application is through the Oriel online portal. This is the UK-wide recruitment portal used for post-graduate specialty training. You will first need to register for an account through their website www.oriel.nhs.uk . Once the programme vacancy window is open then you can access the application form. The application form for General Practice is very factual and requires you to submit your personal details and employment history.

There is a relatively short window (about 3 weeks) to complete the application. I would recommend giving yourself plenty of time to complete the application form as you cannot progress without completing all the sections and there is quite a lot to get through. There is a save function to use as you go along so you do not need to complete it all in one sitting.

REFERENCES

At this stage you need to give the contact details for 3 referees. These need to be your clinical or educational supervisor from your current post, your previous post and the post before that. The requests for references are sent automatically by Oriel once you have inputted their email address. A request for a reference is a very typical task for a supervisor to be asked to complete and most supervisors are happy to fill them out.

It is good practice to ask the referee in person or by email that they are happy to fill out a reference prior to submitting your application. This helps to confirm that you have the correct email address and makes them aware of the impending reference request. It may be many months since you were in that post and they have probably supervised other doctors since so it helps to remind them who you are and gives a positive impression.

An example of a suitable email:

> Dear Dr. Richardson,
>
> I completed an F1 post in Respiratory Medicine between December 2020 and April 2021 and you were my clinical supervisor. I am now in my F2 year and applying for GP training. The application form requires a reference to be completed for this post. Would you be happy if I submitted your name as a referee?
>
> Kind regards,

Some applicants may be concerned about getting a poor reference however the purpose of the referencing is to confirm that you have completed the post that you stated on your application and identify any serious concerns. If there have been concerns that the supervisor thinks should delay training, then they should have already raised with the applicant while on the post. Once referencing is completed and the applicant moves onto the longlisting stage the references do not have further impact on the application.

FOUNDATION COMPETENCIES

As the specialty programme starts at ST1 level the programme requires to see evidence of meeting the competencies of the foundation programme. If you are currently an F2 doctor on the foundation programme then you just need to tell them the name of your foundation school however your place on the programme is conditional on completing foundation training and receiving a Foundation Programme Certificate of Completion (FPCC).

If you are applying to start the programme within 3.5 years after the FPCC was signed, a common scenario if doctors have taken some time working as a locum or abroad following foundation training, then you will need to upload a copy of the certificate to your application form. Those on another UK specialty training programme who are applying for GP specialty training will not need to demonstrate they have achieved foundation competencies as long as they hold a national training number or a deanery reference number as it is assumed that the other specialty training will have assessed for this. This is also true if the applicant has resigned voluntarily from GP specialty training previously.

If none of these apply to you, for example it has been longer than 3.5 years since your FPCC was signed, or you have moved from abroad then you may require a Certificate of Readiness to Enter Specialty Training (CREST). This certificate has to be obtained by demonstrating the foundation competencies during a post of at least 3 months, needs to be signed by a consultant or equivalent and should have been obtained by the time of application.

PREFERENCING

Probably the biggest decision that you need to make at this stage is which of the training programmes you would like to apply for. The application form allows you to rank in order of preference all the GP training programmes in the UK as well as detailing those that you do not want. The reasons for applying to different programmes is very personal but things to consider may be:

Geography – Some applicants may want to be in a part of the country that they are familiar with or have family and friends in. Others may have hobbies that affect their choice, it will be difficult to do much mountain climbing in Norfolk.

Commuting time – Think about whether you would be happy to commute to this area from where you live or whether you would have to move. Also take into consideration traffic volume or whether there are the required public transport links. Sometimes programmes can cover a large area, especially if rural, and you will need to think if you would be happy to travel to any of the practices in that area.

Previous experience – Some doctors want to stay in the areas that they have done previous work or training as they know the hospitals and the local systems. The opposite can also be true where the applicant wants a fresh start or does not think highly of the local services.

Differences between deaneries – although GP training programmes are reasonably homogenous there are differences. For example the East Midlands deanery is offering 24 months in Primary Care whereas the minimum is 18 months.

Targeted Enhancement Recruitment Scheme (TERS) – Some programmes struggle to attract trainees and this is more likely due to them being remote or deprived than the quality of the training programme. In order to make these areas more attractive a scheme was introduced to offer a one-off payment of £20,000 to those that agree to work in these locations.

Opportunities beyond training or medicine – For many it will be too early to be thinking about what to do after training but for some, for example those considering academic work, it may affect their preferences.

Before making the preferences I would recommend looking at the websites for the different deaneries and training programmes as well as doing some research on the local area.

There is a second window to update your preferences from the date of MSRA invitation to 48 hours before the first offers date so there is time to continue thinking about this after completing the initial application.

COMPETITION RATIOS

When preferencing candidates often look at the competition ratios for the different deaneries. This can be a useful tool to aid decision making however needs to be approached with caution and understanding.

A competition ratio is the number of first ranked applicants divided by the number of places. The competition ratios for the round 1 2021 applications are overleaf:

- Round 1 2021
- HEE East Midlands 1.8
- HEE East of England 1.3
- HEE Kent, Surrey & Sussex 1.4
- HEE London 3.2
- HEE North East 1.3
- HEE North West 2.1
- HEE South West 1.5
- HEE Thames Valley 2.3
- HEE Wessex 1.5
- HEE West Midlands 1.8
- HEE Yorkshire and the Humber 1.1
- Health Education and Improvement Wales 1.1
- NHS Education for Scotland 1.9
- Northern Ireland Medical and Dental Training Agency 1.9

As you can see, according to the competition ratios London is by far the most competitive. This is useful as if you were considering applying for the London deanery you will know that you need to put it as your first choice if you want to get a place but may have to consider alternatives if you do not score highly enough.

Other deaneries may have a lower competition ratio but candidates applying to these may face competition from other applicants who put it as a lower preference but did not score highly enough to get into their first choice.

Also when you do preferencing it is the training programme, not just the deanery, that you are choosing. You don't know the competition ratios inside the deaneries. As such some training programmes, for example ones closer to London, may be more competitive than more rural programmes in the same deanery.

Competition ratios also change from one year to the next depending on a few factors such as the number of places and past ratios may not be indicative of the future. In fact places with lower competition ratios in the previous round may become more competitive when you apply because applicants think they stand more chance of getting a place.

In conclusion, GP specialty training is not a competitive enough specialty for competition ratios to matter much. Overall there is not much to be gained from studying them too hard. It is a much better strategy to consider where you want to spend the next 3 years, rank accordingly and do well at the MSRA so that you do your best to guarantee your preferred programme.

OTHER GP TRAINING PATHWAYS TO CONSIDER:

Academic Clinical Fellowships

There are a small number of fellowships that combine specialty training with research training. The academic portion is 25% and therefore would extend training from 3 to 4 years. This may be suitable for those who are considering a career in research alongside general practice. It would be expected that they have shown an interest in academic work prior to applying.

Global Health Fellowships

There are some opportunities for GP trainees to spend some time out of programme working abroad, for example in a rural hospital in South Africa, to develop personal and professional skills. The trainee would then be able to complete their General Practice training on return.

Both of these fellowships have different application processes depending on the region that is being applied to. If they are of interest then further information can be found on the GP recruitment website:
www.gprecruitment.hee.nhs.uk/Recruitment

MULTI-SPECIALTY RECRUITMENT ASSESSMENT (MSRA)

Once you have submitted an eligible application you will be invited to book a place to complete the MSRA via email from Oriel. It is a computer-based assessment that take place at Pearson Vue test centres of which there are locations in many towns and cities in the UK and internationally. There is some provision for alternative arrangements for those unable to attend the centres in exceptional circumstances due to impact from the COVID-19 pandemic.

As the name implies the assessment is used for many different specialties including psychiatry, obstetrics and gynaecology and radiology and therefore the range of topics assessed is broad. This is good for prospective GPs as all the knowledge is likely to have application in future practice. The budding obstetricians having to revise the workings of the prostate may think otherwise.

The assessment consists of a situational judgement paper, that they refer to as professional dilemmas, and a clinical problem solving paper. These are timed individually but are both completed in one sitting. There is an optional 5 minute break between the papers.

As of 2021 there are:
50 questions in the Professional Dilemmas paper for which you are given 95 minutes
97 questions in the Clinical Problem Solving paper for which you are given 75 minutes

The scenarios and problems in the test are aimed to be relevant to a foundation level doctor and can take place in a hospital, general practice or an out-of-hours setting.

The scores from the MSRA are used to determine your ranking and thus whether you have been successful in your application to your chosen programme. Therefore there is great incentive to perform well at the MSRA.

Professional Dilemmas

The aim of this part of the test is to assess judgement in different clinical, and sometimes non-clinical, scenarios. Those that have applied to the Foundation Programme will have completed a situational judgement test at this time and at its core this is similar.

There are two types of question split roughly evenly between:

- Ranking – Rank from most to least appropriate action in response to a particular situation
- Multiple Choice – Choose the 3 most appropriate actions, out of 8, to perform together to most appropriately resolve a situation

As this is a paper to test judgement it will not be possible to revise like a knowledge exam. However, like any test, effective preparation can maximise the marks achieved. Before considering answers, let's first think about what the Professional Dilemmas paper is trying to assess.

There are 3 core target domains:

1) Professional Integrity
2) Coping with Pressure
3) Empathy and Sensitivity

As a doctor these should all be things that we consider ourselves to do well and I'm sure that we can think of real-life dilemmas in our careers where these domains are relevant. It may be on an on-call shift when you get multiple tasks through in succession, or when breaking bad news to a patient or being honest when something does not go to plan. These were all things we faced and acted appropriately and sensitively in response. Unfortunately, the assessors were not there when you demonstrated this and thus the Professional Dilemmas paper is the imperfect way that the MSRA assesses these attributes.

As the professional dilemmas paper is an assessment of decision making it can appear more difficult to revise for than the tests of clinical acumen that we have completed countless times at medical school and beyond. In order to show the assessor your full potential and achieve a high score it would be foolish not to effectively prepare.

There is some subjective judgement when answering these questions however it would be expected that the applicant always acts within the guidance of Good Medical Practice and is able undertake ethical decision making. When working on the wards or in other healthcare settings this will be second nature, and this is why giving the most appropriate answer is often easy. A more thorough understanding of these concepts allows us to disentangle the other options that we are not likely to do in clinical practice.

MEDICAL ETHICS

Most of you will be familiar with the core principles of medical ethics, already having employed the principles throughout your training to date.

When presented with a question on medical ethics, it is essential to think about how the main principles of medical ethics apply.

The main principles of medical ethics are:

Beneficence

The wellbeing of the patient should be the doctor's first priority. In medicine, this means that one must act in the patient's best interests to ensure the best outcome is achieved for them, i.e. 'Do Good'.

Non-Maleficence

This is the principle of avoiding harm to the patient, keeping with the Hippocratic Oath "First do no harm". There can be a danger that in a willingness to treat, doctors can sometimes cause more harm to the patient than good. This can especially be the case with major interventions, such as chemotherapy or surgery. Where a course of action has both potential harms and potential benefits, non-maleficence must be balanced against beneficence.

Autonomy

The patient has the right to determine their own health care. This, therefore, requires the doctor to be a good communicator so that the patient is sufficiently informed to make their own decisions. 'Informed consent' is thus a vital precursor to any treatment. A doctor must respect a patient's refusal for treatment even if they think it is not the correct choice. Note that patients cannot demand treatment – only refuse it, e.g. an alcoholic patient, if deemed to have capacity, can refuse rehabilitation but cannot demand a liver transplant.

There are many situations where the application of autonomy can be quite complex, for example:

- Treating children: Consent is usually required from the parents, although the autonomy of the child is taken into account increasingly as they get older.
- Treating adults without the capacity to make important decisions. The first challenge with this is in assessing whether or not a patient has the capacity to make the decisions. Just because a patient has a mental illness does not necessarily mean that they lack the capacity to make decisions about their health care.

Where patients do lack capacity, the power to make decisions is transferred to the next of kin (or Legal Power of Attorney, if one has been set up).

Justice

This deals with the fair distribution and allocation of healthcare resources for the population. When answering a question on medical ethics, you need to ensure that you show an appreciation for the fact that there are often two sides of the argument. Where appropriate, you should outline both points of view and how they pertain to the main principles of medical ethics and then come to a reasoned judgement. It is important to know that sometimes the beneficence and autonomy may be in conflict. For example, consider a patient that is refusing treatment that could be lifesaving. It is possible that sometimes the patients make decisions that are not correct or in conflict with beneficence duties of a doctor. When faced with such scenarios, try to understand the reasoning of the patient. Is it because of fear, ignorance or something different, for example religious beliefs. If the decisions of the patients are fully informed and the patient has the capacity to make well informed decisions (patient is not confused due to illness/drugs or mental illness) then clinicians must respect the autonomy of the patient.

Further important concepts in medical ethics include:

Consent

This in a way is an extension of Autonomy: patients have the right to first agree (or refuse) to a procedure, treatment or intervention. For consent to be valid, it must be a voluntary informed consent. This means that the patient must have sufficient mental capacity to make the decision and must be presented with all the relevant information (benefits, side effects, and the likely complications) in a way they can understand.

Confidentiality

Patients expect that the information they reveal to doctors will be kept private. This is a key component in maintaining the trust between patients and doctors. You must ensure that patient details are kept confidential. This often comes up in scenarios where relatives may be asking for information about their parent who is a patient (has the patient given you permission to talk to their relative about their condition?) or if a patient/relative tries to have a discussion in the corridor (can you have the discussion in a more private area, less likely to be overheard?). Confidentiality can be broken if you suspect that a patient is a risk to themselves or to others, e.g. terrorism, child abuse, informing the DVLA if a patient is at risk of seizures, road accidents, etc.

MENTAL CAPACITY ACT

The primary purpose of the 2005 act is to govern the decision-making process on behalf of adults who lack the capacity to make decisions for themselves. There are several principles to be aware of:

1. A person must be assumed to have capacity unless proven otherwise.
2. A person is not to be treated as unable to make a decision unless all practicable steps to help them to do so have been taken without success.
3. A person is not to be treated as unable to make a decision merely because they make an unwise decision.
4. An act must be in their best interest.
5. The act must be the least restrictive with regards to the individual's freedoms.

Capacity

Medical capacity arose from the Mental Capacity Act. It's the patient's ability to decide that they can make specific decisions about their care. The capacity is time and 'point' specific, meaning that they may not have the capacity to make complex financial decisions but can take decisions if they would like to have/decline specific treatment.

This can change in time so there may be a time when they have capacity but other times when they don't (even within days or hours, depending on their clinical condition). For example, a patient admitted with a severe infection may not have capacity on their first day in hospital but this may change as they improve with treatment.

When assessing capacity, it is important to know that the individual does not have an underlying mental illness or a reason to compromise their decision-making abilities.

Important things to consider are:

1. Can the patient understand the information?
2. Can the patient retain the information?
3. Can they analyse the information correctly?
4. Can they communicate their choices clearly?

Any deficiency in any of these steps can lead to the patient lacking capacity to make a decision. The understanding of this process is crucial as doctors are often faced with situations where patients may make decisions that are not in keeping with medical advice (e.g. a Jehovah's Witness refusing blood products and having serious blood loss). Carrying out procedures or treatment that directly contravenes a patient's wishes who has capacity is a breach of patient's autonomy, and can be prosecuted.

Doctors should consider a formal mental capacity assessment in the following scenarios:

1. Sudden change in mental status
2. Refusal to treatment, e.g. unclear reason or due to irrational biases/beliefs
3. Known psychiatric/neurological condition
4. People at extreme of ages < 18 years or > 85 years

MEDICAL LAW

Here is a brief overview of some key legal cases and principles that you should familiarise yourself with:

Mental Health Act

This act basically governs how heath care professionals interact with people with mental disorders and their rights to force treatment. The original act was passed in 1983, but there was a significant amendment in 2007.
The most significant components for health professionals are the definition of holding powers, which allow doctors to detain and treat a patient with a mental illness against their will. Most notably, these are the section 5(2) and 5(4) defining doctors' and nurses' duties respectively. Other orders to be aware off are Section 135 (magistrate order) and section 136 (police order), as well as section 2 and section 3 (detention for diagnosis and treatment, respectively).

Data Protection Act

This act gives the GMC power to control how data is collected, recorded and used. Personal data under the act is defined as identifiable information. It's important that data is:

1. Processed fairly and lawfully
2. Gathered for specific purposes.
3. The data is adequate, relevant, accurate and kept up to date

This governs how doctors collect patient information and who they can share this information with. Practical examples are doctors being allowed to break confidentiality for acts of suspected terrorism and road traffic accidents.

Gillick Competence

Children under the age of 18 can consent to treatment if they are able to understand, weigh up, and decide they want the treatment. However, they cannot refuse treatment until they are 18 years old. For children under 18 with no parent/guardian who aren't Gillick competent, you are able to act 'in their best interest'.

Bolam Test

The Bolam test is a legal rule that assesses the appropriateness of reasonable care in negligence cases involving a skilled professional. The Bolam test states "If a doctor reaches the standard of a responsible body of medical opinion, he is not negligent". In order for someone to be shown to be negligent, it must be established that:

1) There was a duty of care
2) The duty of care was breached
3) The breach directly led to the patient being harmed

Euthanasia

Euthanasia is a deliberate intervention undertaken with the express intention of ending a life to alleviate pain and suffering. The two main types of euthanasia are:

- Active Euthanasia: Doctor causes the patient to die, e.g. by injecting poison
- Passive Euthanasia: Doctor lets the patient die, e.g. withdrawing life-sustaining treatment, switch off lifesupporting machines

TIPS FOR ANSWERING PROFESSIONAL DILEMMA QUESTIONS

- Read GMC 'Good Medical Practice' guidance
- Be patient-centred and don't compromise patient safety
- Usually the patient is of primary importance, then your colleagues and then of lowest importance is yourself.
- Maintain honesty and integrity
- Use ethical principles to justify your answer
- Work well in a team

Within the MSRA - there are a number of different question types that you will commonly face. Below, we've provided examples and explanations for each type.

Ranking Questions

In these questions a scenario is given and then 5 possible actions that you can take in response. You need to rank these from most appropriate to least appropriate. It is important to read the question carefully and consider what competency the dilemma is testing.

Example 1:

You are working on a care of the elderly ward and have been asked to insert a naso-gastric tube into Mr Banks, a 90-year-old patient. You are confident in the technique and have done some before. When you go to gain his consent, he tells you he doesn't want the procedure and is 'happy to leave things be'.

Rank in order **the appropriateness of the following actions** in response to this situation (1=Most appropriate; 5= Least appropriate).

A.	Cancel the procedure
B.	Discuss the situation with the consultant
C.	Have a chat with Mr Banks and explain the pros/cons of the procedure so you are sure he is making an informed decision
D.	Proceed with the naso-gastric tube insertion
E.	Explain to the patient that he can change his mind at any time

Answer: CBEAD

This question explores understanding of consent. Although the patient is 90 years old there is nothing to suggest that he lacks capacity. Although we may consider it in his best interests to have the procedure we have to respect the patient's autonomy. However it may be that Mr Banks does not understand fully why he needs the tube therefore **C** is the most appropriate answer. **B** would be the next most appropriate answer as it shows that you have respected Mr Banks autonomy. By talking to the consultant they may be able to think of an alternative or discuss further with Mr Banks. However by this stage of training it would be expected that you would be able to check the patient's understanding and it may waste time to wait for the consultant therefore C is more appropriate.

E shows that you are considering the patient's wishes but does not show any exploration into why he feels this way. It is more appropriate than **A** as it gives Mr Banks the option that he can change his mind again. **D** is the least appropriate answer as it does not respect his autonomy.

Example 2:

You are on ward round with your consultant and a nurse, Shaline. You notice that Shaline is not washing her hands in-between patients. Your hospital has a strict infection control policy that requires you to report her to the infection control nurse on your ward for not following policy.

Rank in order **the appropriateness of the following actions** in response to this situation (1=Most appropriate; 5= Least appropriate).

A.	Tell Shaline she is putting patient safety at risk by not washing her hands in-between patients
B.	Report her to the infection control nurse
C.	Suggest that the infection control team put posters on the wards to remind staff to wash their hands
D.	Ignore the issue
E.	Discuss this at the next MDT when Shaline is present

Answer: ABECD

In this question we need to think about communication between colleagues. It also requires some judgement about following policy. **A** is the most appropriate answer as it pro-actively gives a solution to the ongoing issue. It is expected that you, as a doctor, would be able to take a leadership role on the ward and, politely, confront colleagues. It could be argued that **B** follows the infection control policy more closely however this would be a harsh response without first speaking to the nurse herself as she is likely to be disciplined. **E** offers a poor solution as it does not address the problem directly however it does at least mean that infection control is discussed with Shaline present. **D** is not appropriate and it is negligent to ignore the issue.

Example 3

Your specialty trainee informs you that she was given a ticket by the police yesterday for speeding. She has told the police she was on-call the weekend you were on-call and has asked if you can tell the on-call rota co-ordinator that you have swapped shifts.

Rank in order **the appropriateness of the following actions** in response to this situation (1=Most appropriate; 5= Least appropriate).

A.	Inform your clinical supervisor of the trainee's request, without naming her, seeking his advice on how to proceed
B.	Decline the trainee's request
C.	Explain to the trainee why her request is inappropriate
D.	Inform the police that the trainee was not working on-call at the weekend
E.	Advise the trainee to tell the police the truth about the situation

Answer: EBACD

Situational judgement questions often look at professionalism. **E** would be the best answer as it not only maintains your integrity but shows that you are promoting honesty to your colleague. **B** is the next appropriate as it resolves the problem directly from your side. **A** shows professionalism by speaking to a senior and asking for advice however I am not sure a supervisor will be able to add much to the situation, especially if you do not name them, and it does not immediately deal with the situation. **C** is a response that may be appropriate after completing one of the better responses however one its own does address immediate concerns. **D** is dishonest.

Example 4

You are an FY2 in general practice. A 14-year-old girl presents with a positive pregnancy test and requests an abortion. Her boyfriend is 15 years old. She is not sure of her gestation but has missed at least 2 periods. She asks you not to tell her parents as they are not aware she is sexually active.

Rank in order **the appropriateness of the following actions** in response to this situation (1=Most appropriate; 5= Least appropriate).

A.	Refer her for termination of pregnancy and inform her parents
B.	Phone her parents immediately to gain their consent and raise your concerns
C.	Contact the safeguarding lead as she is having underage sex
D.	Respect her confidentiality, discuss her options and refer for termination
E.	Attempt to persuade her to continue her pregnancy as you are not comfortable with referring her for termination due to your own beliefs.

Answer: DABCE

This tests understanding of consent. A 14 year old can consent to medical procedures, **D** allows her to access a termination while also respecting her wishes to keep this confidential. The other responses are all inappropriate so it can be difficult to assess which is more appropriate. **A** at least accepts that the patient has capacity and refers her for a termination. It does breach confidentiality however which would be unacceptable in this case. **B** does not follow the patient's wishes and incorrectly asks the parents for consent however it does show willing to resolve the situation. **C** does not act to help the patient and underage sex would not be a reason to contact the safeguarding lead unless there was a large age gap or safety concern. **E** is the least appropriate answer as if a doctor has a personal objection to termination of pregnancy then they should refer the patient to a colleague for unbiased advice.

Multiple Choice Questions

These questions require the applicant to choose, from a list of eight, the three most appropriate actions to do in combination in response to a dilemma.

Example 1

You are an FY2 working on the oncology ward. A lady was admitted yesterday with intermittent headaches and nausea. She has a history of breast cancer, and underwent mastectomy and chemotherapy two years ago. An MRI scan of her head shows a brain mass that is very likely to be metastatic breast cancer. However, the formal radiology report is not back yet. When you see the patient later, she nervously asks what the results of the scan were.

Choose the THREE most appropriate actions to take in this situation.

A.	Tell her she has metastatic breast cancer in her brain with an extremely poor prognosis
B.	Tell her a senior doctor will discuss the results with her once the radiology report arrives
C.	Tell her the radiology report has not come back yet
D.	Ask her if she has any family visiting today
E.	Tell her not to worry and everything will be fine
F.	Tell her you will discuss the results with her once the radiology report arrives
G.	Tell her you have seen the scan but are not allowed to tell her
H.	Ask if she has made a will

Answer: CBD

This question assesses how to handle a situation of likely bad news but you have incomplete information. You need to explain to the patient that the report has not come back (C) and that it will be discussed when it arrives. This is better to be done by a senior (B) than yourself. As you think it is likely to be bad news it is good to find out if she has any family visiting (D) as she is likely to need support with the news. The other options will either unduly reassure or worry the patient.

Example 2

You are an FY2 doctor who is on a ward with Stephen, another FY2 doctor. You do not know each other very well but do get along. You have noticed that, recently, Stephen has been losing a lot of weight and does not ever seem to eat anything in public at least. You know that he is very stressed about his upcoming wedding and is struggling with a lot of financial issues. One afternoon, you see him in the hospital café struggling to keep himself up; he seems very tired and keeps leaning on the wall or the tables for support. You know that the afternoon is very busy with ward rounds and patient consultations.

Choose the THREE most appropriate actions to take in this situation.

A.	Ask him how he is coping with the stress lately
B.	Suggest he talks to his consultant about taking the afternoon off
C.	Suggest meeting after work to discuss his problems
D.	Speak to his fiancée about how the wedding is taking a toll on Stephen's health
E.	Ask him if he is okay and get him a chair to sit on
F.	Try to talk to Stephen about why he is not eating and bring up the topic of possibly having an eating disorder
G.	Tell him that you are feeling tired and stressed too
H.	Advise him to go to the emergency department

Answer: ABE

In this question you need to consider the health of not just Stephen but the potential impact this may have on patient safety. Getting him a chair and asking if he is ok is the kind thing to do in this situation (E) and by asking him how he is coping gives him an opportunity to divulge any information on his terms and shows empathy with his situation (A). However telling him you are stressed too is unlikely to help Stephen. It would not be appropriate to speak to his fiancée nor make an assumption that he may have an eating disorder. He has a busy afternoon and patient safety should not be risked with him in his current state. He should talk to his consultant (B) about an afternoon off however going to the emergency department for this condition would waste medical resources.

Example 3

You are an FY2 doctor on your lunch break with your colleague, Kristen, in the hospital cafe. During your break, a young man approaches the both of you. He seems to have been crying. He tells Kristen that he is the son of one of her patients, Mrs Jasdeep. He asks her if she will be alright, but you know that Mrs Jasdeep has been diagnosed with incurable brain carcinoma. He asks when he will find out the diagnosis. Kristen then mutters under her breath 'I cannot even have a peaceful lunch without being interrupted' and continues to eat her lunch. The man seems to have heard her and begins to cry. You must decide what to do.

Choose the THREE most appropriate actions to take in this situation.

A.	Tell Kristen to help the man
B.	Reassure the man that his mother will be ok
C.	Try to calm the young man down
D.	Advise Kristen to eat elsewhere if she wants a peaceful lunch
E.	Tell Kristen, while in front of the relative, that her behaviour is inappropriate
F.	Ask the patient to wait in the relatives' waiting room and that someone will be with him shortly
G.	Tell him that Kristen will speak with him when she has finished lunch
H.	Confirm the relationship of the young man with the patient

Answer: CFH

This question tests your ability to deal with challenging situations while maintaining professionalism. Kristen's comment was inappropriate and unacceptable and this should be fed back to her however not in front of the patient. As the man is upset, you should try and calm him down (C) rather than Kristen. It would be appropriate to confirm his relationship with the patient (H) and ask him to wait in the relatives' waiting room (F) so that someone could speak to him in privacy. This should not be Kristen following her unacceptable comment. Reassuring him that his mother is going to be ok is not ethical.

Example 4

A patient has been prescribed twice the normal recommended dose of a drug by the consultant. The ward nurse points this out to you and queries the dose, as he has not seen this dosage prescribed before. The consultant is currently attending to a patient on a different ward.

Choose the THREE most appropriate actions to take in this situation.

A.	Ask the patient if she knows the reason for the higher dose
B.	Phone the consultant to discuss the dose
C.	Explain to the nurse that the consultant is highly experienced, and that the dose should be administered as prescribed
D.	Advise to not give the dose until it can be discussed with the consultant
E.	Explain that you do not know the reason for the unusual dose, and advise the nurse to seek out the consultant
F.	Speak with the ward pharmacist regarding the dose
G.	Speak with the ward sister about the nurse's actions
H.	Decrease the dose to the usual prescribed dose until you are able to discuss the matter with the consultant

Answer: BDF

This question is about prioritising patient safety. The consultant has responsibility for the prescription and therefore queries should be directed to them (B) however this should be done by yourself and rather than pushed onto a colleague. To maintain safety you should advise that administration of the drug should be held until the dose can be clarified (D). It is good to involve the pharmacist as well as the consultant may not be aware of the correct dosing (F). You should not alter the dose yourself without understanding whether the initial dosing was a mistake. Being able to query prescriptions is important and the nurse's concern should not be dismissed or lead to reporting to his senior.

Clinical Problem Solving Questions

This part of the MSRA test is a test of clinical acumen. There is a broad range of topics that can be tested and a foundation-level of knowledge is expected. This means that if you are applying for the GP specialty programme but have never worked in General Practice you will not be at a disadvantage.

If you have reached this point in medical training you will have passed many exams testing clinical knowledge. You should know the revision techniques that work for you and hopefully you can utilise these for the MSRA too. Remember that when applying for the GP specialty training programme you are competing against competent peers who are also highly skilled at exam taking. Getting higher marks compared to the other applicants is rewarded well in the application process.

The 12 clinical topic areas are:

- Cardiovascular
- Dermatology/ ENT/ Ophthalmology
- Endocrinology/ metabolic
- Gastroenterology/ Nutrition
- Infectious Disease/ Haematology/ Immunology/ Allergy/ Genetics
- Musculoskeletal
- Paediatrics
- Pharmacology & Therapeutics
- Psychiatry/ Neurology
- Renal/Urology
- Reproductive
- Respiratory

The clinical problem solving paper questions should be balanced between these topic areas. These areas cover nearly every field of medicine but this should not come as a surprise. GPs should be prepared for anything and have a wide knowledge base. Some of the groupings seem arbitrary (e.g. Dermatology and ENT) however I think this reflects that foundation doctors are likely to have had less experience in those areas and therefore the test will reflect this in the number of questions on that topic.

Do not fall into the trap of reducing focus on these areas that are grouped. You are likely to have a high knowledge base already in some topics, for example you should have some clinical experience in cardiovascular and respiratory through general medical rotations. This will also be true of the other applicants. Success in the topics that others may be less confident in is an opportunity to elevate your mark above your peers to achieve the best chance of a successful application to your chosen programme.

Also be mindful of potential gaps in your knowledge. You may not have had to think about some topics since medical school. For those who have taken time out of training or been working in a different specialty this may be a long time ago. Guidelines often change and it is important to make sure you are up to date for the test.

When approaching the Clinical Problem Solving paper:

- Leave enough time to prepare – there is too much content that could potentially be tested to leave it all to the last minute – at least 8 weeks of preparation would be recommended
- Play to your strengths – you will have revised successfully for many exams in the past. Think what kind of reviser you are. Some prefer to write notes when revising, others are very visual or prefer auditory techniques. The important thing is recognising how you work and maximising this method.
- Do practice questions – this is a really good way of improving exam technique, testing revised knowledge as well as identifying areas of weakness in our knowledge

- Be careful of just doing practice questions – it may be tempting to just repeat practice questions until your marks improve. This is not a good approach as over time you may be liable to learning the questions rather than knowing the answer. Also, as they do not release many official practice questions to try, there are often differences in style between the practice questions and that of the real exam. Therefore you can leave yourself vulnerable to underperformance.
- Read around topics even if you get practice questions correct – Another temptation when doing practice questions is to assume that you already know a topic when you answer questions correctly. This may be the case however remember that a question will only test a snapshot of knowledge. You may correctly identify the first line medication for hypertension but does this mean that you are adequately prepared when asked about the 2nd or 3rd line treatment when tested?
- Find suitable revision resources – the NICE Clinical Knowledge Summaries are good and have a broad range of topics covered. GP notebook is another free online resource that can be useful. You may be fortunate to have clear, concise notes from medical school to help you revise. Just be aware that guidelines do frequently change and if it has been a few years since graduation then you may need to check these are up to date.

Types of questions

The paper covers five core domains

1) Investigation
2) Diagnosis
3) Emergency
4) Prescribing
5) Management (non-prescribing)

There are two types of question in the Clinical Problem Solving paper:

Type 1: Extended matching

You will be given a list of potential answers and then multiple questions linked to that answer set. Be mindful that potential answers may be used once, not at all or multiple times.

Example 1:

A) Giant Cell arteritis
B) Medication overuse headache
C) Migraine
D) Subarachnoid haemorrhage
E) Tension headache
F) Cluster headache
G) Glioblastoma
H) Myopia
I) Acute sinusitis

For each patient please select the single most likely diagnosis. Answers may be used once, multiple times or not at all.

1. 65 year old male patient experiences a sudden onset severe occipital headache with associated vomiting and neck stiffness. Answer: **D** *This is the typical history of the 'thunderclap headache' that is associated with subarachnoid haemorrhage*

2. 30 year old male patient presents with recurrent left sided frontal headaches with associated eye watering that last approximately 30 minutes. The pain is severe and occurs at the same time every day. Answer: **F** *The short duration and recurrence at the same time daily indicates cluster headache over migraine*

3. 10 year old female patient with episodes of headaches affecting the whole head with associated vomiting and abdominal pain. She is well between episodes. Answer: **C** *Migraine is the most common headache in children. It is often bilateral and they are more inclined to have gastro-intestinal features. We may be concerned about the possibility of Glioblastoma however the child is well between episodes and the question asks for the most likely diagnosis – which in this case is migraine.*

4. 60 year old female patient presents with a one day history of right sided headache. It is not improved with simple analgesia. There is tenderness over the temporal region. Answer: **A** *This is a classical history of Giant Cell arteritis. There may also be associated jaw pain and visual problems.*

Example 2:

A) X-ray
B) MRI
C) DEXA
D) CT
E) PET scan
F) Ultrasound
G) Fluorescein Angiography

For each patient please select the single most appropriate mode of investigation. Answers may be used once, multiple times or not at all.

1. An 89 year old male patient presenting to the Emergency department with a scalp laceration following a fall. She has a background of atrial fibrillation and takes apixaban. **D** *Patients on anticoagulation require an urgent CT scan following a head injury to investigate for intracranial haemorrhage*

2. A 58 year old female patient. She has a background of rheumatoid arthritis and a 40 pack year smoking history. There is concern she may be at risk of a fracture. **C** *A DEXA scan would measure a patient's bone mineral density and help evaluate their risk of osteoporosis.*

3. A 12 year old female patient presents with right leg pain. There is a bony swelling to the distal femur. **A** *The painful bony swelling would be a red flag for osteosarcoma. Although we aim not to expose children to radiation, in this case an urgent x-ray would be indicated.*

4. A 64 year old male patient has abnormal liver function tests found on routine bloods. He is otherwise well and there is no obvious cause from the history. **F** *Of the investigations listed an Ultrasound scan of the abdomen would be the only modality that would give any further relevant information.*

5. A 40 year old patient presents with wrist pain and deformity following a fall onto an outstretched hand. **A** *This is a likely Colles' fracture and would be confirmed on x-ray.*

Type 2: Single Best Answer

In these questions a scenario is given with a list of 5-8 potential answers below. The candidate needs to select the most appropriate answer from the list.

Example 1:
A 60 year old male patient has an average blood pressure of 165/95 following home blood pressure monitoring.

Select the single most appropriate management option from the list below: Select One option only.

A) Furosemide
B) Oxybutinin
C) Ramipril
D) Amlodipine
E) Spironolactone
F) Atenolol

Answer: D
This question tests knowledge of the management of hypertension. A calcium channel blocker is indicated first-line in patients over 55 with stage 2 hypertension.

Example 2:
An 80 year old female patient has become short of breath with associated lip swelling and reduced oxygen saturations following administration of IV Co-amoxiclav. Anaphylaxis is suspected.

Select the single most appropriate initial management option from the list below: Select one option only.

A) Oral Loratidine 10mg
B) IM Hydrocortisone 200mg
C) IM Adrenaline 0.5ml 1:1000
D) IV Adrenaline 10ml 1:10000
E) IV Amoxicillin 500mg
F) IV 0.9% Saline 500ml

Answer: C

Emergency management is one of the core domains tested in the paper. Make sure you know the difference between adrenaline doses required in anaphylaxis and CPR.

Example 3:

A 65 year old female patient presents with 3 weeks of morning stiffness in the neck and shoulders. You suspect polymyalgia rheumatica.

What is the single most appropriate blood investigation to support your diagnosis? Select one option only

A) Urea and electrolytes
B) Calcium
C) Thyroid function tests
D) ESR
E) HbA1C
F) ANA
G) Rheumatoid factor

Answer: D

Inflammatory markers are usually raised in polymyalgia rheumatica therefore ESR would be the correct answer. If you were to review this patient then it is likely that you would perform some of the other tests in the question at the same time however this would be to investigate the differentials rather than support your diagnosis.

Example 4:

A 19 year old female patient presents having had an episode of unprotected sexual intercourse 72 hours prior. She requests emergency contraception but does not want a coil. She has a BMI of 22.

What is the single most appropriate management option?
Please select one option only

A) Ulipristal acetate 30mg
B) Mirena intrauterine device
C) Varenicline 500 micrograms
D) Desogestrel 75 micrograms
E) Misoprostol 400 micrograms

Answer A
Ulipristal acetate (also known by the brand name ellaOne) is the only answer that is used for emergency contraception. Desogestrel and the mirena coil are used for contraception but not in emergencies. Misoprostol is a drug mostly used in medical terminations. Varenicline is used to treat nicotine addiction.

TIPS

Day before the Test

- Make sure that you have familiarised yourself with the tutorial on controls and screen layouts on the Pearson VUE website

The Test

- Keep an eye on time – there are 97 questions to complete in 75 minutes – you have approximately 46 seconds for each question
- Answer every question – there is no negative marking therefore there is no advantage to leaving an answer blank
- Flag questions that you want to spend more time on – The Pearson Vue computer system that you use to complete the test allows you to flag questions as you go through. When you reach the end of the questions you can easily see which ones you need to go back to
- Read the questions carefully – this may seem obvious but is really important as it can be a really easy way to lose marks. Be vigilant for any questions asking for negative e.g. which answer is **not** a cause...
- Look at the demographics - the MSRA is not trying to catch you out and will usually give typical examples rather than red herrings. Think if a potential diagnosis is found more frequently in males or females or the old or the young
- Remember in extended matching questions that answers may be given multiple times or not at all. Don't discount an answer because you have already used it for another question
- If you have not heard of an answer then it is unlikely to be correct. Hopefully if you have adequately prepared then there should not be surprises. As there are multiple choice answers sometimes an obscure one will be added. Do not feel disheartened for not knowing it, it is more likely to be there to catch out guessers. Remember they are testing knowledge at a foundation-level

Overleaf, we have provided a full mock MSRA paper, in line with the current specification. You should only sit this paper only after revising all of the content up until this point in the guide, you are familiar with all of your clinical knowledge, and you can work undisturbed in timed conditions.

MSRA MOCK PAPER

PROFESSIONAL DILEMMAS

Part 1. Ranking

1.	You are working on a busy ward. A locum consultant has just started working with the team the previous day. In the middle of your shift, a patient you are taking bloods from tells you that she heard the new doctor on the phone talking about you in a derogatory way. This is surprising to you as the locum consultant has been nice to you whenever he has spoken to you so far.

Rank in order **the appropriateness of the following actions** in response to this situation (1=Most appropriate; 5= Least appropriate).

A.	Approach the consultant and talk to him about what you were told
B.	Ignore the patient as she is known to spread rumours amongst the ward
C.	Discuss this with another FY2 colleague
D.	Discuss this with your educational supervisor
E.	Ask the patient more about what she heard and what the consultant said

2.	You are attending to a patient on a female psychiatric ward. While taking a history, the patient becomes agitated and holds up a knife, threatening to stab you. You feel threatened.

Rank in order **the appropriateness of the following actions** in response to this situation (1=Most appropriate; 5= Least appropriate).

A.	Hit the panic button and leave the room
B.	Leave the room
C.	Try to de-escalate the situation
D.	Ask one of the nurses to support you
E.	Order her to put the knife down

3.	An 89-year-old, Mr Ratko, is due to be discharged today to a nursing home. He is a long-term patient and requires 24-hour care for a stroke which has left him unable to carry out basic tasks at home. His wife died 20 years ago so he has been living alone with visits from his children. When you see him today, he tells you he has changed his mind and does not want to go to a nursing home.

Rank in order **the appropriateness of the following actions** in response to this situation (1=Most appropriate; 5= Least appropriate).

A.	Ask him why he has changed his mind
B.	Explain that staff in the hospital are too busy to provide him 24-hour care
C.	Explain that a nursing home is better suited to his needs
D.	Tell your consultant that Mr Ratko is unsure about going to a nursing home
E.	Call Mr Ratko's relatives in to discuss his options with him

4.	You are on the ward starting the night shift when you notice an FY2 colleague who is going home, put a list of patient names with notes about diagnosis and management plans in her bag.

Rank in order **the appropriateness of the following actions** in response to this situation (1=Most appropriate; 5= Least appropriate).

A.	Inform your colleague of the breach of confidentiality
B.	Advise your colleague to leave the list in hospital, or destroy it
C.	Report the incident to your consultant the following day
D.	Ask her for the list
E.	Report your colleague to the GMC

5.	You attend a call on the ward about an urgent CT scan. The FY2 has filled out the form but has not put down the cause for the CT and the radiologist is refusing to scan the patient without this information. You know the consultant had asked for it earlier. When you speak to the FY2, she tells you she does not know and walks away.

Rank in order **the appropriateness of the following actions** in response to this situation (1=Most appropriate; 5= Least appropriate).

A.	Call the consultant and explain the situation to him
B.	Ask an available doctor for advice
C.	Ask the radiologist to overlook it as the scan is urgently needed
D.	Ask the radiologist to contact the FY2
E.	Ask the radiologist to contact the consultant

6.	You are an FY2 working on the Emergency Admissions Unit. You are caring for a patient with Multiple Sclerosis who has been admitted with severe dehydration. He is refusing oral or IV fluids and says he wants to die as he is a burden on his family, but he doesn't want them to know he is refusing treatment. He was assessed by liaison psychiatry 2 years ago, who found he did not have any mental health problems such as depression.

Rank in order **the appropriateness of the following actions** in response to this situation (1=Most appropriate; 5= Least appropriate).

A.	Tell the patient that if the family ask directly about his treatment you are duty bound to tell them he has decided to refuse treatment
B.	Encourage the patient to discuss his feelings about MS with his family
C.	Ask liaison psychiatry to assess him again as his mood appears to be very low
D.	Respect the patient's wishes as he is not depressed and his prognosis is poor
E.	Tell the family so that they can speak to him about refusing treatment

7.	You are an FY2 working in outpatient cardiology. You see Boris, who is 56 years old and has recently been diagnosed with hypertension. He does not accept that his high blood pressure could cause heart disease as he 'feels fine' and so will not take the antihypertensives prescribed by the GP. He becomes angry when challenged and admits he has been using homeopathic remedies instead.

Rank in order **the appropriateness of the following actions** in response to this situation (1=Most appropriate; 5= Least appropriate).

A.	Tell Boris there is no evidence for homeopathy so he is being unreasonable
B.	Do nothing, he has the right to refuse treatment and has had it explained before
C.	Explain the consequences of untreated hypertension and its treatment options
D.	Refer Boris back to the GP so they can explain their prescribed treatment again
E.	Advise Boris to see his GP in one month for a repeat blood pressure reading as it is still high today, so he should reconsider taking the prescribed medication

8.	You are an FY2 working on a healthcare of the elderly ward. You were very upset last week as a patient you were particularly fond of died. While you were dealing with the aftermath, another patient's relative asked to speak to you. You explained you would not have time until that afternoon as there had been a death on the ward. The ward sister told you today that the patient's relative has made a formal complaint about your care of their mother, calling you 'inattentive'.

Rank in order **the appropriateness of the following actions** in response to this situation (1=Most appropriate; 5= Least appropriate).

A.	Ask for evidence from witnesses of the encounter
B.	Contact the patient's relative to discuss the complaint
C.	Contact your medical defence union
D.	Collect evidence of your good conduct to send to the GMC
E.	Inform your consultant

9.	You are scheduled to be on call today as an FY2. You are suffering from sinusitis which is causing vertigo. Although you feel well enough to go to work, this morning you do not feel comfortable driving to work due to the vertigo, as you think it will make you unsafe on the roads.

Rank in order **the appropriateness of the following actions** in response to this situation (1=Most appropriate; 5= Least appropriate).

A.	Call in sick
B.	Use public transport to get to work and inform your team why you may be late
C.	Call the team to say you will wait for the vertigo to improve before driving in
D.	Drive anyway as you have a duty to your patients
E.	Make an excuse about your car not working to explain your absence

10.	You are an FY2 working in the emergency department. A patient is brought in by ambulance after having his second tonic-clonic seizure this year. He refuses to stop driving as he is a delivery lorry driver and has a family to support

Rank in order **the appropriateness of the following actions** in response to this situation (1=Most appropriate; 5= Least appropriate).

A.	Write to the patient's GP to get them to persuade him to tell the DVLA
B.	Immediately report the patient to the DVLA without informing him
C.	Write to the patient to remind him of his duty to inform the DVLA
D.	Inform the patient that you are duty bound to contact the DVLA for safety reasons
E.	Only report the patient to the DVLA with his consent

11.	You are an FY2 working on a surgical ward and one of the patients under your care is the uncle of an FY1 working on a medical ward. This FY1 asks you how her uncle is doing so she can report back to her family.

Rank in order **the appropriateness of the following actions** in response to this situation (1=Most appropriate; 5= Least appropriate).

A.	Tell her she should ask the consultant in charge as you are not sure what to say
B.	Tell her all you know about her uncle's surgery and recovery
C.	Say he is fine but you need her uncle's permission before you can tell her anything in more detail
D.	Invite her to join in the handover later today where her uncle will be discussed
E.	Give her his patient ID so she can read the notes on the computer

12.	You have finished a busy shift on the surgical admissions ward. Your colleague, who is due to take over from you, has not arrived yet. It is 15 minutes after the shift has ended and she has just called to say they will be at least 15 more minutes. Handover takes 30 minutes and you have a social engagement of drinks with your friends to attend. This is the first time this has happened to you, what should you do?

Rank in order **the appropriateness of the following actions** in response to this situation (1=Most appropriate; 5= Least appropriate).

A.	Message your friends at the social event explaining you will be late
B.	Make a list of urgent patient cases and outstanding investigations to leave in the general doctors' office after your shift ends
C.	Make a list of urgent patient cases and outstanding investigations to give to your colleague when they arrive
D.	Tell your speciality trainee that you need to leave for a family crisis and brief them on the handover
E.	Message your colleague that you need to leave and if they are late like this it is up to them to call you or find out the patient information from the nurses

13.	You are working in a busy A&E. You take the history of Ms Yee, a 47-year-old patient, with pain in her shoulder and a family history of heart attacks. She asks you tearfully if she is going to die today

Question task e.g. Rank in order **the appropriateness of the following actions** in response to this situation (1=Most appropriate; 5= Least appropriate).

A.	Explain the concept of referred pain and that her passing is a possibility and she should call her loved ones
B.	Soothe her crying and tell her everything will absolutely be okay
C.	Explain that it is a busy day in the ward and her situation is not worth crying over compared to other people you have to attend to
D.	Tell Ms Yee that you must take a thorough history and further tests and examinations must be performed, and a more senior doctor will be able to discuss the outcomes of those with her soon
E.	Tell Ms Yee that you will contact your registrar to discuss the case and explain to her the possible outcomes

14.	During ward round, you encounter a patient who has a skin infection that has seemingly not responded to the initial antibiotics prescribed. Your consultant, Dr Michaels, tells you to prescribe a second antibiotic. When carrying this out the pharmacist informs you that this new drug is not on the hospital formulary and you should not prescribe it because of a risk of antibiotic-resistant bacterial infection developing.

Rank in order **the appropriateness of the following actions** in response to this situation (1=Most appropriate; 5= Least appropriate).

A.	Ignore the pharmacist's advice, prescribe Dr Michaels' request and make a note of it in the patient's notes
B.	Contact Dr Michaels before prescribing anything, to discuss the course of treatment
C.	Ask your speciality registrar to review the patient and make a decision
D.	Prescribe whatever the pharmacist advises
E.	Explain that you are an FY2 doctor, so it would be better for the pharmacist to discuss the situation with Dr Michaels

15.	You are working with an oncology team and see Mr Crookes, a patient who had been treated some years ago for an adenocarcinoma. His symptoms suggest a recurrence and possible metastasis of the cancer and he is under investigation. You are reviewing a nearby patient when Mr Crookes beckons you over and asks if his cancer is back.

Rank in order **the appropriateness of the following actions** in response to this situation (1=Most appropriate; 5= Least appropriate).

A.	Get a colleague to continue taking the observations and take Mr Crookes to a private room and explore his fears
B.	Explain that you do not have his test results, but you will discuss them with him when you do
C.	Explain that you will follow up his test results and get a senior colleague to discuss the results
D.	Tell Mr Crookes he looks well and is going to be fine
E.	Tell Mr Crookes his cancer is likely to have come back based on population statistics

16.	When completing patient notes on a busy ward, you realise you have mixed up the treatment advice plans for two patients, with different conditions, who have been discharged back to their GP. The error was yours and it means each GP will receive a treatment recommendation for the other patient.

Rank in order **the appropriateness of the following actions** in response to this situation (1=Most appropriate; 5= Least appropriate).

A.	Contact the patients to alert them and explain the mix up
B.	Tell the consultant about the mix-up and let them handle it
C.	Ask a fellow FY2 trainee what to do, as they may have done this before
D.	Do nothing as you do not want to get in trouble and the GP will likely recognise the mistake
E.	Adjust the hospital records of the patients as the GP will see the different name and contact the hospital to follow up the correct notes

17.	You see a post on Facebook, where two fellow FY2 colleagues in the same placement are making public and offensive remarks about being "fed up of all the patients at the Royal Free Hospital". They do not appear to be aware of the lack of privacy settings on this post and are disclosing some identifiable patient cases. This is the first time they have ever posted something like this.

Rank in order **the appropriateness of the following actions** in response to this situation (1=Most appropriate; 5= Least appropriate).

A.	Privately message them alerting them to the privacy of their conversation and that it should be taken down
B.	Ask your speciality registrar to have a word with them
C.	Screenshot the post and submit it to the GMC as a complaint
D.	Wait a few days to see if someone else tells them to take the post down
E.	'Like' the post as you want to build rapport with your colleagues

18.	You have joined the paediatrics team and you often work with an FY2 doctor, Lucas. Over the past month you have noticed that Lucas often belittles your professional judgement, interrupts you and disagrees with you. At times this is in front of patients. You are concerned this behaviour is going to continue, or even worsen over time, but you are not sure whether it is just because you are the newest addition to the team.

Rank in order **the appropriateness of the following actions** in response to this situation (1=Most appropriate; 5= Least appropriate).

A.	Start recording and documenting Lucas' behaviour towards you
B.	Ask your registrar what you should do, without naming names
C.	Ask your Foundation Director if you can be moved to a different placement
D.	Try and approach Lucas and discuss how you feel
E.	Wait for 2 weeks to see if time improves the situation

19.	Ms Roach, a 48-year-old lady, has been admitted for investigation due to unexplained feelings of nausea, pain and feeling warm all the time. Her husband comes in with her to the hospital but had to leave after 2 hours for work. He calls frequently to ask for updates on his wife, having been given permission by Ms Roach. On this occasion however, you have just received urine tests with high levels of hCG indicating she is pregnant, which is something she is not aware of yet.

Rank in order **the appropriateness of the following actions** in response to this situation (1=Most appropriate; 5= Least appropriate).

A.	Tell Mr Roach it would be best for him to speak to Mrs Roach directly about her condition when she is free to talk
B.	Tell Mr Roach that tests are being run to investigate and explain the symptoms
C.	Tell Mr Roach you need to speak to a senior colleague about the case before speaking to him
D.	Tell Mr Roach that you need to obtain Mrs Roach's permission again, and you will call him back
E.	Tell Mr Roach about the positive result on the urine test

20.	A nurse comes up to you voicing her concerns that Mr Edu, an elderly patient, does not fully understand why he is going into theatre. You see from his notes that your colleague, an FY2 doctor, has obtained the consent forms for this minor operation.

Rank in order **the appropriateness of the following actions** in response to this situation (1=Most appropriate; 5= Least appropriate).

A.	Call the theatre to cancel the operation
B.	Ask the specialty trainee to check Mr Edu's understanding of the operation
C.	Tell Mr Edu to speak to someone to withdraw his consent until it is explained to him adequately
D.	Speak to Mr Edu and check his understanding of the operation
E.	Tell the consultant your concerns regarding consent for the operation

21.	Henry is an 8-year-old boy who was admitted in the morning as he was recently diagnosed with a tumour in his pancreas. He has come back today for further tests and you advised his family that he would have an MRI and PET scan in a few hours' time. The parents took time off work and have been waiting in the hospital with Henry. 3 hours later, the radiology department tells you the scan will not be performed until tomorrow as they had some emergency cases and have a backlog of patients. You tell Henry's parents and his mother starts to react angrily towards you in front of other patients.

Rank in order **the appropriateness of the following actions** in response to this situation (1=Most appropriate; 5= Least appropriate).

A.	Tell the parents that the information you gave them earlier was correct at the time and you could not have predicted this
B.	Tell the mother to lodge a formal complaint if she wants to
C.	Apologise for the delay and hear out the mother's concerns in a private setting
D.	Politely explain that emergency cases need to be seen before Henry
E.	Shout back that it was the radiology department's fault not yours, and she should take up her complaints with them

22.	One of your patients has COPD and has been in hospital for 4 weeks. He is desperate to go home and has been told he can go home providing he wears an oxygen mask hooked up to an oxygen tank. He is very excited about the prospect of going home. He confides in you a 'secret' that he does in fact smoke - you know this to be a direct contraindication for the oxygen therapy at home as there is a risk of an explosion.

Rank in order **the appropriateness of the following actions** in response to this situation (1=Most appropriate; 5= Least appropriate).

A.	Sign him up to a smoking cessation programme
B.	Tell the patient he cannot go home now unfortunately
C.	Discuss the reason why you cannot permit oxygen therapy due to the smoking hazards with the patient
D.	Get the ward nurse to tell him why he cannot go home as you do not want to disappoint him
E.	Tell the patient not to smoke when he goes home and pretend he never told you that he does

23.	You are working on an ENT ward that conducts many research projects and clinical trials. The department is often in the newspapers regarding such achievements. You overhear an elderly patient telling his daughter that he is scared his confidential information will be made public due to research and will be free for all to see.

Rank in order **the appropriateness of the following actions** in response to this situation (1=Most appropriate; 5= Least appropriate).

A.	Ignore the patient as it was a private conversation you overheard
B.	Tell the daughter his information will not be used without his permission
C.	Tell a nurse what you overheard and ask her to reassure the patient
D.	Reassure the patient his information will not be used without his expressed permission
E.	Ask the patient why he has confidentiality concerns and what they are

24.	While working on a busy ward, a senior nurse comes up to you to complete forms for tests for a patient you have never seen before. This will take some time as you would have to familiarise yourself with their drug chart, history and admission. Your team is about to begin a ward round. This will discuss all the most recent patients admitted and you ought to attend.

Rank in order **the appropriateness of the following actions** in response to this situation (1=Most appropriate; 5= Least appropriate).

A.	Complete the task and catch up with the ward round later
B.	Explain to the nurse that you have to attend the round and will do the task straight after
C.	Tell the nurse you have done the task but actually do it when you are free
D.	Tell the nurse you are busy and to ask you later
E.	Shout at the nurse that you are busy and to get someone else to help

25.	You are the FY2 on the cardiology ward. Your consultant is currently not in hospital and your registrar is busy in an outpatient clinic. Suddenly, a patient develops severe shortness of breath. You suspect this is flash pulmonary oedema. You have never treated this before, but you have learnt the theory.

Rank in order **the appropriateness of the following actions** in response to this situation (1=Most appropriate; 5= Least appropriate).

A.	Call the registrar, then assess the patient and begin treatment
B.	Assess the patient and start basic treatment according to protocols
C.	Call the registrar, then wait until he arrives to begin treatment
D.	Ask a fellow FY2 to come with you to assess the patient and start basic treatment
E.	Leave the ward to go to the registrar's outpatient clinic

Part 2: Multiple Choice scenarios

26.	You are working in A&E and attend to Ben, a 5-year-old child with autism who can communicate only through sign language. He has come in with his mother who looks tired. You take them to a side room to examine Ben. Upon taking a history you find that Ben has had abdominal pain since the morning and has not eaten properly or opened his bowels for two days. You start to examine Ben and the mother nods off. As you examine him, you notice bruises on his arms and chest.

Choose the THREE most appropriate actions to take in this situation.

A.	Wake the mother and ask her about the bruises
B.	Call social services immediately
C.	Call a senior and get some advice on the matter
D.	Look at previous records to see if these bruises have been noted before or if there is any record of suspected abuse
E.	Report the mother to the police
F.	Do a full assessment of the child
G.	Get a second opinion of the bruises
H.	Contact another family member of the child

27.	An elderly patient on the ward has been admitted with delirium secondary to a UTI. At lunch you are in the canteen, when you hear some nurses who work on the same ward talking about her. They are mocking her quite loudly and mention her name a few times. People at neighbouring tables can hear them and look uncomfortable. On the far side of the canteen you spot the patient's husband sitting alone looking visibly upset at the conversation.

Choose the THREE most appropriate actions to take in this situation.

A.	Ignore the situation; the patient doesn't know
B.	Report the incident to the ward sister
C.	Tell the nurses that they are breaking confidentiality and demonstrating a lack of professionalism.
D.	Initiate disciplinary action
E.	Monitor the nurse's behaviour over the next week
F.	Speak to your educational supervisor about this
G.	Tell the patient about the incident
H.	Reassure the neighbouring customers

28.	You are working on an orthopaedic ward. After attending to a patient, you feel nauseated and make your way to the toilet where you throw up. Earlier in the day you had eaten a chicken sandwich that had left your stomach feeling a little unsettled. You had ignored it and had come into work as the ward was understaffed. You do not have a fever or pain and feel much better after you throw up.

Choose the THREE most appropriate actions to take in this situation.

A.	Go home without telling anybody
B.	Inform HR so they can organise a locum to cover for you the next few days
C.	Inform your team of which patients haven't been seen
D.	Take a culture and send it to the lab for further investigation
E.	Drink some water
F.	Take cultures from every patient you came into contact with that day
G.	Tell your educational supervisor that you will not be in for a few days
H.	Take a few days off without telling anyone

29.	You are working on an orthopaedic ward when you see a patient, who has just had surgery on her hip, walking around pushing the food tray beside her bed. She should not be mobilising without the proper support of a Zimmer frame and a physiotherapist. When she sees you, she smiles and tells you proudly that she's up and about a day after her surgery. When you ask how she got out of bed, she tells you that a nurse helped her out and gave her the food tray to push around. The nurse left about 15 minutes ago and has not returned.

Choose the THREE most appropriate actions to take in this situation.

A.	Tell her you don't have time to look after her and that she should be in bed
B.	Take her back to bed and explain why she can't mobilise yet and why she needs to rest her hip
C.	Tell her that she'll be able to mobilise when the physiotherapist comes to see her
D.	Ask her to rest her hip
E.	Leave her once she's at the bed and carry on with your work
F.	Answer any questions she has
G.	Tell her she shouldn't leave the bed
H.	Ask her to call a nurse if she wants to walk around and go to the toilet

30.	While in the morning briefing on the paediatric ward, you notice your FY1 colleague Michael, come in a few minutes late with red eyes. He looks slightly unfocussed. When briefing ends, as Michael takes a pen out of his pocket, a small packet of white powder falls out and he quickly puts it back in his pocket. He looks up and catches your eye but leaves before you can say anything. At lunch, Michael corners you in the empty staff room and asks you what you saw.

Choose the THREE most appropriate actions to take in this situation.

A.	Tell the truth about seeing the packet of white powder
B.	Lie and tell him you saw nothing
C.	Tell him you are going to report him to the GMC
D.	Lie about what you saw, but report him to the consultant at the end of the day
E.	Ask him what was in the packet
F.	Tell him you'll speak to him later
G.	Refuse to answer him
H.	Try to de-escalate the situation by calming Michael down and getting him to step away from you

31	Mr Hammon, a 96-year-old man, comes in at the end of your A&E shift with a high fever and marked confusion. He is brought in by his neighbours. They have known him for a long time and tell you that he has been living alone since his wife died a few months ago. One of his children, a son, lives in Hong Kong. A CT scan is performed that shows lesions on the brain, suspected to be metastases secondary to lung cancer. The fever is due to a UTI. The neighbours approach you to speak about the patient's condition.

Choose the THREE most appropriate actions to take in this situation.

A.	Ask the neighbours how long they've known Mr Hammon
B.	Give them general updates like "Mr Hammon is feeling better today."
C.	Ask them if they are aware of any pre-written/agreed documents in which Mr Hammon gives his consent for his neighbours to be involved in his care
D.	Check Mr Hammon's notes for any documents which may indicate previous decisions taken about his care
E.	Ask the neighbours to see if they can get in touch with the son in Hong Kong
F.	Do not interact with the neighbours at all
G.	Discuss this situation with the team
H.	Discuss the issue in the next MDT

32	You are helping in the breast clinic. Just before you are about to start the consultant brings an A-level student into the room and asks if they can sit in with you. They are on work experience.

Choose the THREE most appropriate actions to take in this situation.	
A.	Meet the patient at the door and inform them that you have a student inside
B.	Ask the patient to sit on the bed so you can examine them
C.	Start the consultation
D.	Invite the student to ask a few questions
E.	Introduce the patient to the student
F.	Invite the student to examine the patient
G.	Make no effort to introduce the student
H.	Gain the patient's consent to have the student present during the consultation

33.	You are an FY2 working on a healthcare of the elderly ward. A 4th year medical student is attached to you. She asks if she can catheterise a patient. She has done male catheterisation many times before and can talk you through the steps.

Choose the THREE most appropriate actions to take in this situation.

A.	Gain consent from the patient and let the medical student proceed
B.	Let the medical student catheterise the patient
C.	Clerk another patient as the student catheterises the patient
D.	Observe the student as she catheterises the patient
E.	Do some paperwork as the student carries out the procedure
F.	Explain to the patient that a medical student is going to catheterise her
G.	Talk the student through the steps
H.	Ask the student to observe you

34.	You are on your break and walk in on your registrar crying in the staff room. When you ask him what happened, he tells you that his wife left him yesterday and he hasn't been able to focus today, so much so, that he prescribed the wrong drug for a patient who had a severe anaphylactic reaction. The patient has now filed a complaint form against him and is threatening to sue. Your registrar says he feels hopeless and despairing.

Choose the THREE most appropriate actions to take in this situation.

A.	Reassure him
B.	Tell your consultant that you think he needs extra support
C.	Tell him he needs to forget what happened and carry on
D.	Continue with your work and leave him to deal with his emotions
E.	Suggest that he takes a few days off
F.	Ask him if he's willing to apologise to the patient for his mistake
G.	Discuss the issue with another FY1 colleague
H.	Offer to talk to the patient about what happened

35	A patient comes into the haematology clinic complaining that he's been waiting for an hour to be seen. You apologise for running late and ask him why he's here. The patient is angry and tells you that it's in the notes and that you should have read it beforehand, so he doesn't repeat himself. He demands another doctor.

A.	Refuse to do the clinic again
B.	Discuss what happened with your educational supervisor
C.	The next time you do the clinic, ensure that you explain history taking to all the patients you see
D.	Discuss what happened with your consultant
E.	Reflect on what happened
F.	Use this as a teaching point for history taking to medical students
G.	Ask the patient to apologise to you
H.	Email the patient to apologise for the issue again

36	A recent complaint by a patient has led to a newspaper investigation into the hospital. Melissa has read some articles and tells the doctor she wishes to be treated at a different hospital as she believes she would be better cared for elsewhere.

Choose the THREE most appropriate actions to take in this situation.

A.	Tell her that the newspaper articles are wrong
B.	Assure her that the staff make every effort to provide quality service
C.	Tell Melissa that you will read the articles yourself
D.	Ask Melissa why she thinks this
E.	Allow Melissa to go to a different hospital
F.	Call the newspaper company and tell them to stop the investigation
G.	Tell Melissa that every hospital has their faults
H.	Promise Melissa that she would be better cared for than others

37	You are an FY2 doctor working in A&E. A woman comes with bruising. The triage nurse recognises her as she has been to A&E several times recently. She suspects domestic violence and informs you. However, the woman says she has fallen down the stairs.

Choose the THREE most appropriate actions to take in this situation.

A.	Review the bruises again to see if they seem to be that obtained from falling from the stairs
B.	Ask her to tell you the truth
C.	Ask her if she fears anyone at home
D.	Mention other domestic abuse patients that have also been helped
E.	Promise her that nothing will go wrong
F.	Ask her if there are any children at home who could also be suffering from the abuse
G.	Refer her to social services immediately
H.	Ask the nurse if she is confident that this patient had come to A&E several times before

38	You are an FY2 who is working under Mr. Sanders, a general surgeon. Your cousin is due to be operated on by Mr. Sanders to remove a painful abscess. She is nervous about the operation and asks you what you think about Mr. Sanders. You know that Mr. Sanders is a very good surgeon but is often late when seeing patients on wards. Hence, he is often rushed and flustered when speaking to them before operations, which can make them lose their trust in him. Recently, Mr. Sanders has reported you to your supervisor for not taking history from a patient properly. You must decide what to say to your cousin.

Choose the THREE most appropriate actions to take in this situation.

A.	Becky should tell her that Mr. Sanders is very competent and totally trustworthy
B.	Tell her nothing will go wrong
C.	Tell her Mr. Sanders can seem flustered by that should not affect his ability to perform the surgery well
D.	Say nothing
E.	Tell her she has no choice but to do the surgery so she should not be picky
F.	Tell her the truth about his tardiness
G.	Tell her not to worry
H.	Talk about the competence of Mr. Sanders and omit the truth about his punctuality

39	You join your consultant and two other junior doctors on ward rounds. A patient, Miss Khan, has been diagnosed with a rare condition that is critical and requires surgery. Miss Khan is afraid of having an operation and asks for a second opinion. The consultant, a leading expert on the patient's condition, tells Miss Khan that 'there isn't time for a second opinion' as any delay would put her life at risk. You get on well with the patient and have previously spent a lot of time answering her questions as she was being diagnosed. The patient is very frightened and looks like she is about to cry.

Choose the THREE most appropriate actions to take in this situation.

A.	Bring the patient case up in the next meeting so everyone is aware of the importance of patient autonomy
B.	Reassure Miss Khan that the consultant is competent and a leading expert in this field
C.	Look online for evidence of Miss Khan's claims about the operation
D.	Calm Miss Khan down
E.	Immediately take the consultant aside to discuss allowing a second opinion
F.	Reassure Miss Khan that the surgeries at the hospital are usually successful
G.	Ask Miss Khan what her fears are
H.	Seek advice from another senior doctor who has some knowledge in the field

40	You and Kate are both FY2 doctors working in A&E. When you arrive for the evening shift, Kate does a brief handover, giving you a stack of patient charts. Kate describes some details of the patients' condition, then says that she needs to run, since she has an urgent family matter to attend to at home. As Kate heads out of the ward, you check the patients' charts to find that several of the files contain no notes. Some of the information was filled in when the patients were admitted into A&E, but nothing has been updated since then. A large majority of the notes are also illegible.

Choose the THREE most appropriate actions to take in this situation.	
A.	Immediately try to contact Kate to call her back
B.	Run after Kate
C.	Inform Kate that her notes are illegible
D.	Try to make sense of the notes
E.	Ask another junior about the notes
F.	Ask your senior doctor for advice
G.	Ask nurses if they can make sense of the notes
H.	Tell Kate the next morning that she should improve her handwriting

41	You, an FY2 doctor, are filling in on the ward for another clinician who left on annual leave the day before. You approach the bed of an elderly patient, Mrs Tessephine, who is being handed some tablets and water by a male nurse. Mrs Tessephine says that she is glad to see you. She points to the nurse and says that this man is making her uncomfortable, calling him an immigrant whilst doing so. She then goes on to throwing the tablets on the floor and says she will not take anything that is given to her by 'people who have invaded my country'.

Choose the THREE most appropriate actions to take in this situation.

A.	Tell the patient that this is not how she should behave in a hospital
B.	Tell the nurse that he is an embarrassment to the hospital
C.	Tell the patient that she is being unfair on the nurse
D.	Tell the nurse that maybe he should wait outside while you convince the patient to take the tablets
E.	Ask the patient why she feels this way
F.	Tell the hospital chairman of the nurse's behaviour
G.	Reassure the patient about the competence of the hospital staff members
H.	Persuade the patient to take the tablets

42	You walk into the ward supply cupboard on your night shift. You see an FY1, Lila, sleeping on the floor of the supply cupboard, using her coat as a pillow. You also sees a bin bag filled with some of her belongings. Lila explains that she has been kicked out of her apartment and needs a place to stay just for one night, since her friend has kindly decided to lend her a room after that. It is a busy night and more staff members are bound to walk into the supply cupboard to find her. You are aware that Lila's financial situation is not the best at the moment.

Choose the THREE most appropriate actions to take in this situation.

A.	Tell Lila that she should be ashamed of herself
B.	Ask Lila to start tutoring part time to earn more cash
C.	Seek advice from a mutual friend
D.	Ask Lila if this is why she has been in a bad mood all week
E.	Ask Lila why she has been kicked out of her room
F.	Offer Lila some cash to get a room for the night at a local hotel
G.	Ask Lila if she would like to stay at your flat for the night
H.	Tell Lila that sleeping in the supply cupboard can be an interference considering how often staff members might want to get something from there tonight

43	You are an FY2 doctor working in A&E. Ms Jacqueline presents with a wrist injury, however she is intoxicated and is clearly annoyed with the waiting list. She shouts at one staff member, telling him that he is not doing his job properly and demanding to know how many people are before her in the queue. She is also shouting rudely at the other patients. On one occasion, she shouts at one Indian family, 'These kinds of people just live off benefits, and shouldn't be here taking the treatment I paid for'.

Choose the THREE most appropriate actions to take in this situation.

A.	Ask the patient to leave
B.	Tell the patient she will not be treated if she continues to shout like this
C.	Tell the patient that the hospital does not tolerate such crude behaviour
D.	Try to calm the patient down
E.	Ask the patient if she would like to discuss anything privately
F.	Tell the patient how many people there are before her in the queue
G.	Bring the patient aside and tell her that the hospital does not tolerate such discrimination
H.	Remind her that she is in a hospital and tell her to drink some water

44	You and Kieran are FY2 doctors. Kieran walks into A&E for his night shift and ou smell alcohol on his breath. It is a very busy night and you notice that he seems a little disorientated by the number of people in the ward. You are also aware that Kieran has been having some financial problems as well as some problems at home with his family. He has just been called by his consultant to assist her with a patient.

Choose the THREE most appropriate actions to take in this situation.

A.	Offer to get Kieran a cab home
B.	Ask Kieran if he has a place to stay for the night
C.	Tell Kieran he has to tell his consultant about his condition
D.	Ask Kieran if he signed the hospital guidelines
E.	Tell Kieran what is he doing is inappropriate
F.	Ask Kieran if he is okay
G.	Tell Kieran that, if he has been drinking, then it would be best if he does not see patients
H.	Ask Kieran if he would like to sit down

45	A 55-year old alcoholic is admitted in the afternoon with delirium tremens after stopping drinking a few days ago. One afternoon, you are called to see him as he has become very aggressive and is demanding to be allowed home. He is confused about the date, shouting that it is 1987 and he has a job interview to get to. As you arrive on the ward, he punches one of the nurses. He is also threatening nearby patients who are watching him, some of whom seem very uncomfortable and scared.

Choose the THREE most appropriate actions to take in this situation.

A.	Sedate the patient
B.	Ask the nurses to call the police
C.	Ask the nursing staff to call security
D.	Transfer him to another facility
E.	Attempt to talk to the patient and try to calm him down
F.	Ask your colleagues to restrain the patient
G.	Ask the nurse who was punched if he is okay, making sure the injury is not severe
H.	Reassure the patient about the competence of the staff

46	You and Jennifer are FY1 junior doctors and have been friends since school. When you walk into the supply cupboard one day, you see Jennifer filling a rucksack with bags of IV fluid. However, Jennifer asks you not to tell anyone about it and says that these are supplies for a charity hospital in Zimbabwe.

Choose the THREE most appropriate actions to take in this situation.

A.	Contact the GMC
B.	Let Jennifer continue as it is for a good cause
C.	Check the stock of IV fluid so there is enough for the ward
D.	Tell Jennifer that she should not be taking supplies from the ward
E.	Advise Jennifer to speak with HR if she wants to organise a charity donation
F.	Get your rucksack so Jennifer can take more bags of IV fluid
G.	Inform Jennifer that you will have to speak to the consultant if she does not stop
H.	Give Jennifer some cash as a donation to the hospital in Zimbabwe

47	Wanda is a patient who has been in hospital for a few weeks recovering from a post-surgical infection. When her consultant was supposed to meet her to discuss her recovery with her, he had to leave urgently to answer his bleep call. You are a junior doctor. Wanda asks you on your ward rounds why she is still in hospital since she is desperate to leave that night since it is her grandson's birthday.

Choose the THREE most appropriate actions to take in this situation.

A.	Complete her discharge paperwork
B.	Explain that only a senior doctor can make the decision to discharge
C.	Try and answer any questions that Wanda may have to the best of your ability
D.	Tell her the consultant is doing something more important currently
E.	Try and contact the consultant to find out if he can review the patient
F.	Let Wanda leave but tell her she must come back in the morning
G.	Ignore Wanda's question
H.	Ask the ward sister if she is ready for discharge

48	You are an FY2 working on-call for the respiratory team. Your consultant and registrar are visiting a nearby elderly care home to see some patients there and will be back in another half hour. Whilst doing paperwork, you receive a call from your mother that your grandmother is in A&E as she has had a heart attack. You are very upset by this news and want to go and visit her.

Choose the THREE most appropriate actions to take in this situation.

A.	Leave and go to visit your grandmother
B.	Hand your on-call bleep to the other FY2 on the ward and ask them to cover
C.	Wait half an hour until your consultant returns to inform her that you are leaving
D.	Leave your bleep at reception for the registrar to collect on their return
E.	Handover unfinished jobs to another doctor on the ward
F.	Hand your on-call bleep to the surgical on-call doctor
G.	Complete your shift and then go and visit your grandmother
H.	Take your bleep with you to A&E as it is in the same hospital and you can answer it

49	A patient, Mrs Simmons, is due to be discharged today, back home. Her daughter approaches you in the afternoon and asks you to assess her mother as she is complaining of right arm weakness. When you assess her mother, she presents with significant arm weakness on the right.

Choose the THREE most appropriate actions to take in this situation.

A.	Explain that the discharge paperwork has been completed so she has to go home
B.	Come back in an hour to see if it has improved
C.	Inform the consultant
D.	Document in the notes so it can be reviewed on the morning ward round
E.	Ask the physio to see the patient
F.	Let the ward sister know she will no longer be discharged today
G.	Complete a full neurological examination
H.	Request an urgent MRI scan

50	You are working on a care of the elderly ward. A patient with a tremor is given a cup of hot coffee. He is unable to drink coffee without help. Whilst you are clerking another patient with the registrar, you notice that he tries to drink the coffee and spills it all over the table. The doctor speaking to him gets him some tissues to clean the mess and then places the cup on top of the tissues. She then leaves.

Choose the THREE most appropriate actions to take in this situation.

A.	Continue clerking your patient
B.	Shout to the patient to not pick up the cup as he may spill again
C.	Sit with the patient and help him drink his coffee
D.	Clean the mess up properly
E.	Ask a nurse to help him with his coffee
F.	Write 'No Hot Drinks' on a board behind the patient's bed
G.	Let the other doctor know she left the patient in a poor state
H.	Get the patient a fresh cup of coffee as he spilled his first

CLINICAL PROBLEM SOLVING PAPER

Pharmacology and Therapeutics

1. A 48 year old female patient was recently diagnosed with hypertension and has been started on ramipril.

Which of the following is the SINGLE most common side effect of ramipril? Select ONE answer only.

A) Rash
B) Dyspepsia
C) Shortness of breath
D) Diarrhoea
E) Cough

2. A 56 year old female patient who was recently prescribed carbimazole for hyperthyroidism presents with a sore throat and fever.

Which of the following investigations is the SINGLE most appropriate initial investigation? Select ONE answer only:

A) TFTs
B) FBC
C) Throat swab
D) Blood cultures
E) UEs

3. A 56 year old male patient has been commenced on warfarin after a mechanical valve replacement. He is counselled regarding medications which may affect his INR (International Normalised Ratio).

Which ONE of the following medications is most likely to increase his INR? Select ONE answer only:

A) Carbamazepine
B) Phenytoin
C) Rifampicin
D) Sodium valproate
E) Phenobarbitone

Medication side effects

A) Methotrexate
B) Amlodipine
C) Ciclosporin
D) Gold
E) Bendroflumethiazide
F) Doxycycline
G) Amoxicillin
H) Simvastatin
I) Bisoprolol

For each question, which of the above medications is the most likely to have caused the side effect? Select ONE option only for each question, each option may be selected once, more than once or not at all:

4) A 54 year old female patient experiencing swollen gums and excessive hair growth after being initiated on treatment for rheumatoid arthritis. (C)

5) A 42 year old male patient on treatment for psoriatic arthritis is reviewed for gradually worsening shortness of breath. His chest X ray reveals fibrotic changes. (A)

6) A 22 year old male patient presents to his GP after he develops a rash on his face following sun exposure. He has recently been started on a new medication. (F)

7) A 72 year old female patient who has recently been discharged from hospital after suffering a myocardial infarction. She has follow up bloods done with her GP a week later which reveals an acute kidney injury and hyponatraemia. (E)

8) A 63 year old male with a history of atrial fibrillation has recently been started on a medication following a transient ischaemic attack. He presents to his GP with muscle aching. (H)

Gastroenterology

9. A 76 year old female patient with a previous history of open cholecystectomy is admitted to hospital with abdominal pain and vomiting. She last opened her bowels two days ago and denies passing flatus. On examination her abdomen is slightly distended and diffusely tender with absent bowel sounds.

Which of the following is the SINGLE most likely diagnosis? Select ONE answer only:

A) Constipation
B) Acute pancreatitis
C) Small bowel obstruction
D) Ischaemic bowel
E) Appendicitis

10. A 28 year old male patient presents with a four week history of bloody diarrhoea and weight loss. After review by gastroenterology and subsequent colonoscopy he is diagnosed with Ulcerative Colitis.

Which ONE of the following is a common extra-intestinal manifestation of Ulcerative Colitis? Select ONE answer only:

A) Uveitis
B) Eczema
C) Glaucoma
D) Interstitial lung disease
E) Type II Diabetes Mellitus

11. A 28 year old male patient presents to his GP with a three month history of fatigue, weight loss and diarrhoea. You suspect a diagnosis of Coeliac Disease.

Which ONE of the following investigations is most likely to confirm this diagnosis? Select ONE answer only:

A) Stool microscopy and cultures
B) Faecal calprotectin
C) H. pylori serology
D) Barium swallow
E) Tissue transglutaminase antibody assay

12. A 56 year old female patient with a history of gall stones presents to the Emergency Department unwell with abdominal pain and vomiting. She is not jaundiced. On examination she is noted to have severe epigastric tenderness, her blood pressure is 110/76 mmHg, temperature is 37.5 C and her heart rate is 115. Bloods reveal an ALT of 175 iU/L, Bilirubin 20 micromol/L, ALP 32 iU/L and an Amylase of 400 U/L.

Which ONE of the following is the most likely diagnosis? Select ONE answer only:

A) Cholecystitis
B) Pancreatitis
C) Cholangitis
D) Gastritis
E) Duodenal ulcer

13. A 75 year old male patient with a history of hypertension and GORD presents to his GP with a one month history of worsening acid reflux, decreased appetite and weight loss. There has been no change in bowel habit or vomiting. He takes amlodipine 5mg and lansoprazole 15mg.

Which ONE of the following options is the most appropriate next management step? Select ONE answer only:

A) Organise a chest X ray
B) Helicobacter pylori serology
C) Refer for urgent endoscopy
D) Increase lansoprazole to 30mg
E) Urea breath test

Causes of Jaundice

A) Pancreatic cancer
B) Biliary colic
C) Acute cholangitis
D) Liver cirrhosis
E) Sickle-cell anaemia
F) Hepatocellular carcinoma
G) Gilbert's syndrome
H) Primary sclerosing cholangitis

For each patient, which of the above options is the most likely diagnosis? Select ONE option only for each question, each option may be selected once, more than once or not at all:

14) A 19 year old female patient from Jamaica presents with recurrent episodes of abdominal pain. The most recent episode was following an upper respiratory tract infection. She has previously been noted to be jaundice and her mother suffers from the same condition. (E)

15) A 24 year old female patient suffers from mild recurrent episodes of jaundice, but is otherwise well. During a most recent episode of jaundice, her bilirubin was 70 micromol/L. All other liver functions tests were within normal range. (G)

16) A 72 year old male patient presents to his GP with a two week history of painless jaundice. He has been experiencing night sweats and has lost 10kg of weight in the last two months. (A)

17) A 42 year old female patient presents to the Emergency Department with a one day history of right upper quadrant pain, fevers and jaundice. (C)

18) A 62 year old male patient with a history of alcohol dependence presents to the Emergency Department confused, jaundiced with abdominal distension. On examination he is noted to have signs of ascites and asterixis. (D)

Cardiovascular

19. A 65 year old female patient with no significant medical history was recently been diagnosed with hypertension by her GP. After discussion of the risks and benefits of treatment, it was decided that drug therapy would be trialled. She presents a week later with bilateral ankle swelling. She is otherwise well.

Which is the SINGLE most likely cause for her symptom? Select ONE answer only:

A) Congestive cardiac failure
B) Amlodipine
C) Ramipril
D) Nephrotic syndrome
E) Lymphoedema

20. A 42 year old female patient presents with retrosternal chest pain that is worsened on taking a deep breath in and relieved by sitting forward. She has no breathlessness, nausea, palpitations or syncope. An ECG shows widespread ST segment elevation in most leads and a Troponin I done three hours after the onset of pain is normal.

Which is the SINGLE most likely diagnosis? Select ONE answer only:

A) Myocardial infarction
B) Pulmonary embolus
C) Endocarditis
D) Pericarditis
E) Costochondritis

21. A 70 year old female patient with a background of type II diabetes, hypertension and a 20 pack-year smoking history presents to his GP with intermittent left calf pain. The pain starts after walking 20 metres and is relieved by rest. On examination his left leg and foot appear normal in colour however there is a slightly delayed capillary refill time and he has absent peripheral pulses.

What is the SINGLE most likely diagnosis? Select one answer only

A) Venous insufficiency
B) Deep vein thrombosis
C) Intermittent claudication
D) Spondylolisthesis
E) Thrombophlebitis

22. A 68 year old female patient with a history of hypertension and previous myocardial infarction presents to her GP with exertional breathlessness worsening over two months. She has no cough or fever. On examination she is noted to have ankle oedema and auscultation of the chest reveals bi-basal fine inspiratory crackles.

Which ONE of the following is the most likely diagnosis? Select ONE answer only:

A) Pneumonia
B) Chronic obstructive pulmonary disease
C) Asthma
D) Congestive cardiac failure
E) Lung cancer

23. When giving adrenaline to a patient in cardiac arrest, what is the correct dose and route of administration? Select ONE answer only from the options below:

A) 1mg given as 1ml of 1:1000 IM
B) 1mg given as 10mls of 1:10,000 IV
C) 0.5mg given as 10mls of 1:500 IV
D) 1mg given as 1ml of 1:1000 IV
E) 0.5mg given as 5mls of 1:10,000 IM

Dermatology / ENT / Eyes

24. A 22 year old female patient presents to her GP with a rash that has been present for several months. It presents as groups of intensely itchy and fluid filled blisters on her extensor surfaces. A diagnosis of dermatitis herpetiformis is suspected.

Dermatitis herpetiformis is most commonly associated with which of the following? Select ONE answer only:

A) Coeliac disease
B) Ulcerative colitis
C) Intra-abdominal carcinoma
D) Irritable bowel disease
E) Crohn's disease

25. A 56 year old smoker with a history of dyspepsia presents to his GP with a 3 weeks history of a hoarse voice. Examination of his chest and throat is normal.

What is the most appropriate next step in the management of this patient? Select ONE answer only:

A) 2 week wait referral for suspected cancer
B) Start lansoprazole 30mg OD
C) Refer for endoscopy
D) Phenoxymethylpenicillin 500mg QDS
E) Refer to stop smoking services

26. A 75 year old male patient presents with pain, redness and decreased vision in their left eye. You suspect a diagnosis of closed angle glaucoma.

Select the SINGLE medication which should be avoided in this patient. Choose one option only.

A) Carbamazapine
B) Amitriptyline
C) Pregabalin
D) Gabapentin
E) Nefopam

27. An 82 year old male patient presents to his GP with a slowly enlarging lesion on his right cheek. On examination the lesion is noted to be 6mm in diameter, has rolled pearly edges and surface telangiectasia with central ulceration.

Which ONE of the following is the most likely diagnosis of this lesion? Select ONE answer only:

A) Malignant melanoma
B) Basal cell carcinoma
C) Squamous cell carcinoma
D) Actinic keratosis
E) Keratotic horn

28. A 48 year old female patient presents to her GP with worsening hearing loss over a period of three months. There are no abnormalities on otoscopy. When performing Weber's test the sound lateralises to the right ear. In Rinne test bone conduction is greater than air conduction in the right ear. In the left ear air conduction is greater than bone conduction.

Which of the following options best described the type of hearing loss described? Select ONE answer only:

A) Conductive hearing loss right ear
B) Conductive hearing loss left ear
C) Sensorineural hearing loss right ear
D) Sensorineural hearing loss left ear
E) Bilateral sensorineaural hearing loss

Dizziness

A) Meniere's disease
B) Vestibular neuronitis
C) Cerebellar stroke
D) Acoustic neuroma
E) Otitis media
F) Benign positional paroxysmal vertigo
G) Orthostatic hypotension
H) Multiple sclerosis

For each patient, which of the above options is the most likely diagnosis? Select ONE option only for each question, each option may be selected once, more than once or not at all:

29) A 78 year old male patient with a history of atrial fibrillation experiences sudden onset constant vertigo which is so severe that he cannot walk. There is no hearing loss. On examination he has nystagmus. (C)

30) A 64 year old female patient presents to her GP with intermittent episodes of vertigo and nausea. She explains that her symptoms are worse on movement, particularly when turning over in bed. (F)

31) A 75 year old female patient recently diagnosed with hypertension presents with intermittent episodes of dizziness on standing which improve after a few seconds. She has no hearing loss or nausea. (G)

32) A 24 year old male patient with a history of Neurofibromatosis Type II presents to his GP with gradual onset left sided hearing loss, tinnitus and vertigo. Ear examination is normal bilaterally. (D)

33) A 40 year old female patient presents with a history of intermittent episodes of vertigo each lasting one hour, associated with intermittent tinnitus, aural fullness. She is found to have sensorineural hearing loss. (A)

Infectious disease / haematology / immunology / allergies / genetics

34. A 19 year old male patient presents to his local walk in centre with a week history of sore throat, fever and fatigue. On examination he has bilateral tonsillar enlargement and some cervical lymphadenopathy. He is given a course of amoxicillin and a day later presents to his GP with a widespread non-blanching maculo-papular rash.

Which of the following is the most likely diagnosis? Select ONE answer only:

A) Meningitis
B) Tonsillitis
C) Acute lymphocytic leukaemia
D) Glandular fever
E) Guttate psoriasis

35. A 32 year old male patient is investigated after having been found to have hypertension and microscopic haematuria. He is diagnosed with polycystic kidney disease. His father is affected by the same condition and his mother is neither affected nor a carrier.

Which of the following options best describes the genetic transmission of this form polycystic kidney disease? Select ONE answer only:

A) Autosomal dominant
B) X-linked recessive
C) Autosomal recessive
D) Multi-allelic
E) X-linked dominant

Causes of anaemia

A) Iron deficiency
B) Thalassaemia
C) Pernicious anaemia
D) Anaemia of chronic disease
E) Alcohol
F) Acute lymphoblastic leukaemia
G) Bowel cancer
H) Sickle cell anaemia

For each patient, which of the above options is the most likely diagnosis? Select ONE option only for each question, each option may be selected once, more than once or not at all:

36) A 42 year old female patient presents to her GP with fatigue. Bloods results show a macrocytic anaemia and further testing reveals low B12 and intrinsic factor antibody is positive. (C)

37) A 48 year old female patient presents to her GP with fatigue and heavy menstrual bleeding. Blood results show a microcytic anaemia. (A)

38) A 74 year old male patient presents with a four month history of altered bowel habit, weight loss and fatigue. Blood results show a microcytic anaemia. (G)

39) A 24 year old female patient from Greece presents with a six month history of fatigue and worsening breathlessness. Blood tests reveal a microcytic anaemia with normal ferritin. (B)

40) A 12 year old female patient presents with a two week history of intermittent fevers, sore throat and raised lymph nodes. Blood tests reveal anaemia and low white blood cell counts. (F)

Neurology / psychiatry

41. A 23 year old female patient is reviewed by an optometrist due to some blurring of vision and loss of colour vision in her left eye. The optometrist suspects optic neuritis.

Optic neuritis is most commonly associated with which of the following diagnoses? Select ONE answer only:

A) Retinal detachment
B) Encephalitis
C) Multiple sclerosis
D) Trigeminal neuralgia
E) Myaesthenia Gravis

42. A 72 year old female patient with a history of polymyalgia rheumatica presents to her GP with a three hour history of a new left sided headache. This is associated with pain in the jaw on chewing and some visual disturbance. On examination she is noted to have tenderness over the left temple.

Which ONE of the following is the most likely diagnosis? Select ONE answer only:

A) Cluster headaches
B) Migraine
C) Giant cell arteritis
D) Trigeminal neuralgia
E) Tension headache

43. A 65 year old female patient with Parkinson's Disease presents to her GP with nausea, vomiting and diarrhoea. Her GP suspects a viral gastroenteritis and decides to prescribe an antiemetic.

Which of the following medications would be the most appropriate to prescribe? Select ONE answer only:

A) Chlorpromazine
B) Cyclizine
C) Metoclopramide
D) Promethazine
E) Prochlorperazine

44. During an admission on a psychiatry ward, a 35 year old male patient is started on Olanzapine as part of his treatment for schizophrenia. Three days after initiation of treatment he develops confusion, rigidity and a fever. His heart rate is recorded as 144 bpm and his blood pressure is 192/112 mmHg.

Select the most likely cause of his presentation from the following. Select ONE answer only:

A) Sepsis
B) Encephalitis
C) Neuroleptic malignant syndrome
D) Mania
E) Extra-pyramidal side effects of olanzapine

45. A 65 year old male patient with a diagnosis of paranoid schizophrenia who has been stable on haloperidol for a number of years is reviewed by his GP. He is noted to have involuntary repetitive movements of his arms and repetitive lip smacking and grimacing. The GP suspects tardive dyskinesia.

Which one of the following statements regarding tardive dyskinesia is true? Select ONE answer only:

A) There is a higher risk of tardive dyskinesia with typical vs atypical antipsychotics
B) Tardive dyskinesia is more common in males
C) There is usually rapid resolution of symptoms with the withdrawal of the drug responsible for symptoms
D) The risk of tardive dyskinesia decreases with the duration of treatment
E) The abnormal movements are usually present during sleep

46. An 82 year old female patient with no significant medical history is reviewed on the orthopaedic ward following a fall and fractured neck of femur which had been fixed in theatre the day before. She presents as acutely confused with visual hallucinations and paranoia.

Select the most likely cause of her presentation. Select ONE answer only:

A) Lewy-body dementia
B) Alzheimer's disease
C) Acute delirium
D) Bipolar disorder
E) Transient ischaemic attack

47. A 52 year old female patient presents to her GP with a 2 day history of a sharp, shooting pain across her right cheek and jaw which she describes as shock-like. The episodes of pain last only a few seconds but are occurring frequently and are usually triggered by eating, talking and light touch to the area.

Which one of the following is the most likely diagnosis? Select ONE answer only:

A) Temporomandibular joint dysfunction
B) Temporal arteritis
C) Trigeminal neuralgia
D) Migraine
E) Cluster headaches

48. A 62 year old male patient with a history of hypertension and peripheral vascular disease presents to his GP after experiencing temporary loss of vision in his left eye earlier on that day. The visual loss is describes as sudden in onset, affecting all of his vision and lasted 15 minutes before resolving completely. He now feels completely well. Cranial nerve examination and fundoscopy is normal.

What is the most likely diagnosis? Select ONE answer only from the following options:

A) Central retinal vein occlusion
B) Transient ischaemic attack
C) Retinal detachment
D) Migraine
E) Acute angle glaucoma

Musculoskeletal

49. A 76 year old female patient presents with a 6 week history of pain and stiffness around his shoulders and hips associated with fatigue. His GP suspects a diagnosis of polymyalgia rheumatica (PMR).

Which one of the following investigation results is consistent with a diagnosis of PMR? Select ONE answer only:

A) An X ray showing osteoarthritic changes in the shoulder and hip joints
B) Raised serum alkaline phosphatase (ALP) levels
C) Raised erythrocyte sedimentation rate (ESR)
D) DEXA scan showing reduced bone density around the shoulders and hips
E) Positive HLA-B27 antibodies

50. A 69 year old male patient with a history of prostate cancer treated 2 years ago with radical prostatectomy presents to his GP with acute lower back pain associated with decreased sensation and power in his left leg.

Select the SINGLE most appropriate management option from the list below. Select ONE answer only:

A) Arrange X ray lumbar spine
B) Referral to physiotherapy
C) Arrange emergency admission
D) Referral to urology
E) Advise analgesia with naproxen and codeine

51. A 52 year old male patient with a history of poorly controlled diabetes and diabetic nephropathy presents with a two day history of a hot, swollen and tender right foot. On examination his first MTP joint is noted to be affected. His current GFR is 32 mL/min/1.73m^2. A diagnosis of gout is suspected.

Select the most appropriate initial therapy from the list below. Select ONE answer only:

A) Naproxen
B) Celecoxib
C) Prednisolone
D) Allopurinol
E) Colchicine

Endocrinology

52. A 40 year old female patient presents to her GP with a several month history of fatigue, lethargy, central adiposity and hair loss. On examination she is noted to have purple abdominal striae, a fatty hump between her shoulders and proximal muscle weakness.

What is the SINGLE most likely diagnosis from the list below. Select ONE answer only:

A) Cushing's syndrome
B) Autoimmune hypothyroidism
C) Addison's disease
D) Conn's disease
E) Type II Diabetes Mellitus

53. A 19 year old male patient with presents to the emergency department with a one day history of abdominal pain and vomiting. He has recently been experiencing increased thirst, weight loss and increased nocturnal urinary frequency. On examination he is noted to be hypotensive, tachycardic and tenderness over the epigastrium. His blood glucose is 32 mmol/L.

Select the SINGLE most likely diagnosis from the list below:

A) Gastroenteritis
B) Hypercalcaemia
C) Diabetic ketoacidosis
D) Pancreatitis
E) Duodenal ulcer

54. A 52 year old lorry driver has been recently been diagnosed with Type II Diabetes by his GP.

Which of the following agents is least appropriate to be started due to the risk of hypoglycaemia. Select ONE answer only:

A) Metformin
B) Empaglifozin
C) Sitagliptin
D) Gliclazide
E) Liraglutide

55. A 38 year old female patient presents to her GP with palpitations and anxiety. Upon further questioning she reveals that she has been losing weight despite eating normally, has been experiencing insomnia and has been more sweaty than usual. On examination she is noted to have a heart rate of 110 bpm, is normotensive, has a tremor and bilateral proptosis.

Which of the following investigations is most likely to confirm the diagnosis? Select ONE answer only:

A) Urinary catecholamines
B) Rheumatoid factor
C) Bone profile
D) Dexamethasone suppression test
E) Thyroid function tests

Electrolyte abnormalities

A) Hyperkalaemia
B) Hypokalaemia
C) Hypernatraemia
D) Hyponatraemia
E) Hypercalcaemia
F) Hypocalcaemia
G) Hypomagnesemia
H) Hypermagnesemia

For each patient, which of the above options is the most likely diagnosis? Select ONE option only for each question, each option may be selected once, more than once or not at all:

56) A 62 year old male patient with a history of prostate cancer presents to the emergency department with confusion, generalised pain and nausea and vomiting. His wife notes that he has recently been drinking more water and urinating more frequently.

57) A 79 year old female patient with a history of hypertension who takes bendroflumethiazide presents with worsening confusion and lethargy.

58) A 62 year old male patient with a history of hypertension presents to hospital unwell after a week of diarrhoea. An ECG shows tall tented T-waves and widening of the QRS complex.

59) A 68 year old female patient with a history of surgically managed thyroid carcinoma presents with muscular aches and pains. On examination she is noted to have some paraesthesia in her hands and feet. Her parathyroid hormone levels are noted to be low.

60) A 40 year old female patient with a history of bipolar disorder treated with lithium presents to hospital following a seizure. Her family note that she has been increasingly confused over the last two weeks and has been urinating up to 15 times a day.

Paediatrics

61. A 2 year old boy is seen in the GP Out of Hours Centre with a two day history of cough and mild fever. On examination he looks generally well and has no signs of respiratory distress. His chest is clear with good bilateral air entry, however you note a barking cough. His SpO2 is 98% and his temperature is 37.9 C.

Which of the following is the most likely diagnosis? Select ONE answer only:

A) Whooping cough
B) Bronchiolitis
C) Inhaled foreign body
D) Croup
E) Epiglottitis

62. A 4 year old girl is seen by her GP with a four days history of rash and sore throat. On examination she is well, her throat is clear and you note some erythematous macules and papules with a central vesicle over her legs, hands and lesions in her mouth. You suspect a diagnosis of hand, foot and mouth disease.

Which of the following organisms is responsible for this presentation? Select ONE answer only:

A) Parvovirus
B) Coxsackie A virus
C) Respiratory syncytial virus
D) Papillomavirus
E) Streptococcus pneumoniae

63. You are seeing a 2 year old child with Down's syndrome on the paediatric ward after he was admitted for observation after a seizure.

Which ONE of the following is typically associated with a diagnosis of Down's syndrome? Select ONE answer only:

A) Early-onset dementia
B) Increased muscle tone
C) Small tongue
D) Increased risk of solid tumours
E) Decreased risk of cardiovascular disease

64. A 1 year old boy presents to the Emergency Department with 24 hour history of intermittent episodes of distress and vomiting. On review the child appears unwell and a sausage-shaped right sided abdominal mass can be palpated. Upon inspection of the nappy you note a redcurrant-jelly like stool.

Which ONE of the following is the most likely diagnosis? Select ONE answer only:

A) Hirschsprung's disease
B) Appendicitis
C) Constipation
D) Pyloric stenosis
E) Intussusception

Lower limb issues in children

A) Slipped capital femoral epiphysis
B) Perthe's disease
C) Transient synovitis
D) Septic arthritis
E) Reactive arthritis
F) Chondromalacia patellae
G) Osgood-Schlatter's disease
H) Ewing's sarcoma

For each patient, which of the above options is the most likely diagnosis? Select ONE option only for each question, each option may be selected once, more than once or not at all:

65) An 11 year old boy presents to his GP with worsening right hip pain. On examination he is noted to be overweight and there decreased internal rotation and flexion of the hip. (A)

66) A 2 year old girl is seen in the emergency department with a two day history of fever and new limp. On examination she is unable to walk and her right hip is flexed and abducted. She has a temperature of 38.6 C. (D)

67) A 14 year old girl presents to her GP with a two month history of worsening left knee pain which is stopping her from competing on her school's athletic team. On examination there she is noted to have tenderness and swelling at the tibial tubercle. (G)

68) A 13 year old boy presents to his GP with worsening pain on his lower leg, particularly at night. This has been associated with fatigue and intermittent fevers. On examination he is noted to have a bony swelling distal to the knee. (H)

69) A 16 year old girl presents with a two day history of right knee pain and swelling. She is otherwise well and is not pyrexial. She was treated for a urinary tract infection one month ago. (E)

Renal / Urology

70. A 55 year old male patient with a background of alcohol dependence presents to the Emergency Department with a two day history of severe intermittent left loin pain radiating to his groin associated with some episodes of vomiting. He has had no dysuria, no increased urinary frequency and no visible haematuria. He is opening his bowels normally. On examination he is apyrexial with normal blood pressure and heart rate. His urine dip is positive only for blood.

Which ONE of the following is the most likely diagnosis? Select ONE answer only:

A) Oesophageal varices
B) Pyelonephritis
C) Ureteric colic
D) Testicular torsion
E) Diverticulitis

71. A 73 year old female patient has had routine blood tests performed for an annual health check. Her eGFR is 55 ml/min. A repeat test three months later shows no change in her eGFR. She is diagnosed with Chronic Kidney Disease (CKD).

Which stage of CKD does this lady have? Select ONE answer only:

A) Stage 1
B) Stage 2
C) Stage 3a
D) Stage 3b
E) Stage 4
F) Stage 5

72. A 78 year old male patient with a background of hypertension and diabetes has bloods done after an episode of gastroenteritis. This reveals an Acute Kidney Injury (AKI).

Which of the following medications is most likely to have contributed to this? Select ONE answer only:

A) Amlodipine
B) Metformin
C) Paracetamol
D) Ramipril
E) Atorvastatin

Testicular problems

A) Testicular torsion
B) Hydrocele
C) Varicocele
D) Epidydimo-orchitis
E) Inguinal hernia
F) Testicular cancer
G) Epidydimal cyst
H) Squamous cell carcinoma of the scrotum

For each patient, which of the above options is the most likely diagnosis? Select ONE option only for each question, each option may be selected once, more than once or not at all:

73) A 32 year old male patient presents to his GP due to problems with fertility. On examination of his testicles he is noted to have left sided scrotal swelling that feels like a "bag of worms". (C)

74) A 19 year old male patient presents to the emergency department with a two hour history of sudden onset right testicular pain which radiated to his abdomen. On examination his right testicle is noted to be elevated and exquisitely tender. There is no redness, swelling or warmth of the testicle. (A)

75) A 19 year old male patient presents to the emergency department with a four day history of worsening right sided testicular pain. He has had a green penile discharge and on examination his right testicle is swollen, warm and tender to touch. (D)

76) A 76 year old male patient presents with a one month history of painless left sided scrotal swelling. On examination he is noted to have a large non-tender left sided scrotal swelling which has a cough impulse. You cannot palpate above the swelling. (E)

77) A 16 year old male patient presents to his GP with a four month history of right scrotal swelling. On examination he has a large, fluctuant and non-tender scrotal swelling that transilluminated when a pen torch is held to it. (B)

Reproductive

78. A 23 year old female patient who is currently 6 weeks pregnant presents to the emergency department with abdominal pain and vaginal bleeding. You suspect an ectopic pregnancy.

Which ONE of the following is NOT associated with an increased risk of ectopic pregnancy. Select ONE answer only:

A) Pelvic inflammatory disease
B) Previous ectopic pregnancy
C) Endometriosis
D) Polycystic ovarian syndrome
E) Smoking

79. A 19 year old female patient presents to her GP for her routine contraceptive review. She is currently taking the oral combined contraceptive.

The risk of developing which of the following cancers increases with the use of the combined oral contraceptive? Select ONE answer only:

A) Endometrial
B) Ovarian
C) Bowel
D) Cervical
E) Lung

80. A 28 year old female patient with a history of irregular periods presents to her GP with reduced menstrual frequency over the past six months. She also notes recent weight gain and complains of facial hirsutism.

Which of the following diagnoses is the most likely? Select one answer only:

A) Type II Diabetes Mellitus
B) Polycystic ovarian syndrome
C) Hypothyroidism
D) Cushing's disease
E) Ovarian tumour

81. An 18 year old female patient presents to the sexual health clinic with malodorous vaginal discharge. Swabs are taken, microscopy reveals clue cells and cultures grow Gardnerella Vaginalis.

What is the diagnosis? Select ONE of the following answers:

A) Candidiasis
B) Gonorrhoea
C) Trichomoniasis
D) Bacterial vaginosis
E) Chlamydia

Breast problems

A) Fibroadenoma
B) Breast abscess
C) Mastitis
D) Ductal ectasia
E) Mammary duct carcinoma
F) Nipple candidiasis
G) Blocked milk duct
H) Paget's disease of the nipple

For each patient, which of the above options is the most likely diagnosis? Select ONE option only for each question, each option may be selected once, more than once or not at all:

82) A 42 year old female patient presents to her GP with a hard, fixed and painless right breast lump which is associated with blood stained nipple discharge. There is also a mass in the right axilla. (E)

83) A 37 year old female patient who is 2 weeks post-partum and breast feeding presents with flu-like symptoms and a painful left breast. Her left breast is noted to have a wedge-like area of warmth and redness. There is no focal lump. (C)

84) A 24 year old female patient presents with a left breast lump that has been present for two weeks. It is firm, smooth, non-tender and high mobile. There are no skin changes and no axillary masses. (A)

85) A 62 year old female patient presents with a red scaly rash on her right nipple and areola. There is evidence of some ulceration on the nipple and on examination a lump is noted. (H)

86) A 46 year old female patient presents to the emergency department unwell with a painful swollen lump in her left breast. The lump is extremely tender to palpation and the overlying skin is hot and erythematous. (B)

Respiratory

87. A 22 year old female patient with a history of asthma presents to the Emergency Department acutely short of breath. She is struggling to speak in full sentences and on auscultation of her chest you note that she has a bilateral wheeze. Her SpO2 is 93%, her pulse is 112 and her PEF is 30% of predicted value. She stabilises after receiving oxygen and a salbutamol nebuliser.

Which ONE of the following options is the next most appropriate step in her management? Select ONE answer only:

A) Discharge with a course of oral steroids
B) Discharge with a course of oral antibiotics and steroids
C) Admission to hospital
D) Monitor for an hour and if still stable discharge
E) Liaise with GP to organise an asthma review

88. A 43 year old female patient presents to the Emergency Department acutely short of breath with pleuritic chest pain. She has a raised D-Dimer and a subsequent CT Pulmonary-Angiogram (CTPA) shows a right pulmonary artery embolism.

Which ONE of the following is a risk factor for developing a pulmonary embolism. Select ONE answer only:

A) Female sex
B) Progesterone only contraceptive
C) Alcohol intoxication
D) Factor V Leiden
E) Distal radial fracture

89. A 36 year old male patient who returned from Bangladesh six months ago presents to his GP with fatigue, persistent cough, weight loss and night sweats. He has been previously fit and well and is a non-smoker. A chest X ray shows an opacity in his right upper lobe.

Which of the following is the most likely diagnosis? Select ONE answer only:

A) Community acquired pneumonia
B) Lymphoma
C) Lung cancer
D) Tuberculosis
E) Asthma

90. A 69 year old male patient presents to his GP with a chronic cough and increasing shortness of breath. He has smoked 10 cigarettes a day for 40 years.

In pack years, what has been his lifetime smoking exposure? Select ONE answer only:

A) 10 pack years
B) 20 pack years
C) 30 pack years
D) 40 pack years
E) 50 pack years

91. An 30 year old male patient presents to his GP with shortness of breath. He is a non-smoker. Spirometry is performed and shows an obstructive pattern and a chest X ray shows signs of hyperinflation and multiple bullae. He is diagnosed with emphysema.

Which of the following is a risk factor for the development of emphysema? Select ONE answer only:

A) Alcohol
B) Leflunomide
C) Asthma
D) Alpha-1 Antitrypsin
E) Intravenous drug use

92. A 68 year old female patient with a background of COPD presents to A&E with increasing wheeze over the last few weeks, and with a slightly purulent cough that she hasn't been able to shake. Her observations on arrival are: HR 80, BP 137/93, Sats 89%, RR 26, Temp 37.9. She has undergone an A through E assessment. You have been asked to help stabilise her.

Which ONE of the following options is the most appropriate first step in her management? Select ONE answer only:

A) Liaise with GP to discuss possible diagnosis of COPD
B) Carry out bloods and arterial blood gas
C) Commence sulbutamol nebulisers
D) Perform further history
E) Obtain a chest x-ray

Investigations in breathlessness

A) Chest X ray
B) Spirometry
C) High resolution CT
D) CTPA
E) BNP
F) Echocardiogram
G) FBC
H) Troponin
I) Fractional exhaled nitric oxide (FeNO) test
J) ECG

For the following cases, which of the above is the most appropriate investigation?
Select ONE option only for each question, each option may be selected once, more than once or not at all:

93) A 63 year old male patient with a forty pack year smoking history presents to his GP with worsening breathlessness over a period of one year. He has no cough or weight loss. Auscultation of his chest reveals some widespread fine crepitations. A recent chest X ray in the emergency department was clear. (B)

94) A 72 year old female patient with a history of previous myocardial infarction presents to her GP with gradually worsening breathlessness over a period of four months, especially on lying flat. She has had associated ankle swelling. (E)

95) A 69 year old smoker presents to his GP with a three week history of cough and an episode of haemoptysis. (A)

96) A 62 year old ex-miner presents to his GP with a worsening history of breathlessness over a period of three months associated with a cough. He has had no haemoptysis or weight loss. On examination you note some clubbing of the nails and some coarse crackles on his chest. A recent chest X ray showed some small round nodular opacities. (C)

97) A 52 year old female patient who recently underwent knee surgery presents to the emergency department with sudden onset chest pain and breathlessness. She is noted to have an SpO_2 of 91% and her heart rate is 123. (D)

END OF TEST

PROFESSIONAL DILEMMAS ANSWER KEY:

1. EADBC
2. ABDCE
3. ADECB
4. ABDCE
5. AEDBC
6. BCDAE
7. CEDBA
8. ECDAB
9. BCAED
10. DBACE
11. CADBE
12. ACBDE
13. DEABC
14. BECDA
15. CBAED
16. ABCED
17. ABCDE
18. DBAEC
19. DBACE
20. DBECA
21. CDABE
22. CBDAE
23. EDCBA
24. BADEC
25. DBACE
26. ADF
27. BCH
28. EBC
29. DBC
30. HAE
31. CDE
32. AHE
33. ADF
34. ABE
35. DEC
36. BCD
37. BFC
38. CGF
39. DHG
40. ACF
41. EHG
42. HGF
43. DFE
44. FGC
45. CEG
46. CEG
47. BEC
48. ABE
49. CGH
50. DEG

PROFESSIONAL DILEMMAS WORKED SOLUTIONS:

1. Answer:	EADBC This question assesses your ability to cope with difficult situations. **E** is the most appropriate, as by obtaining more information, you may be able to work out whether this patient is lying or not. **A** ensures that you sort the problem out immediately. If what the patient has told you is true, you will be able to discuss this with the consultant and iron out your differences. You could discuss this with your educational supervisor (**D**) to get some advice on the matter as they are impartial to the situation and have a duty of confidentiality, but this wouldn't solve the issue. **C** isn't ideal as you don't want to replicate what the consultant is doing by spreading gossip. **B** is also not a good option. You should try and investigate the matter further, as it could potentially harm your reputation on the ward. If the consultant is speaking to you in front of patient's, it may make them doubt you or worry about the professionalism of the staff on the ward.

2. Answer:	ABDCE This is a dangerous situation and you must ensure that you are safe. Hitting the panic button will call for support and leaving the room takes you out of danger almost immediately (**A**). Terminating the interview and leaving the room gets you out of danger but doesn't call for the support you may need (**B**). Calling for a nurse may help as nurses deal with situations such as these, but in this case, you are just putting another person in potential danger (**D**). This is a heated situation and you have to ensure your own safety first (**C**). Ordering the patient to put the knife down will probably make her angrier (**E**).

3. Answer:	ADECB This question assesses patient centred focus, so you must understand why Mr Ratko has changed his mind (**A**). As a patient he has autonomy to make decisions but as a doctor, you also have to utilise your time and space on the ward effectively. Mr Ratko does not need any more treatment beyond what the nursing home can offer but there must be a reason he is hesitant about going. The consultant is in charge of the patient and has agreed the discharge so they need to be kept up to date about what is happening to make any future decisions (D). The family needs to be involved only if the patient consents (**E**). There is no indication they were involved in any previous decisions. Telling Mr Ratko that the nursing home is more suitable to his needs and that the staff are too busy undermines Mr Ratko's confidence in the staff and fails to acknowledge that his wishes have changed (**C and B**).

4. Answer:	ABDCE Your colleague is breaking confidentiality as patient lists are not meant to be taken outside of the hospital. It is important you deal with this situation before your colleague leaves (**A**). Advising your colleague to destroy the list without an explanation may mean she repeats the action (**B**). Asking your colleague for the list, ensures that it does not leave the hospital, but it does not mean that your colleague is aware of her mistake and will not do it again (**D**). **C** does not deal with the situation immediately and unnecessarily involves another person when this could have been dealt with there and then. **E** is completely inappropriate as your colleague's behaviour has not warranted being reported to the GMC.

5. Answer:	AEDBC This question assesses your ability to work under pressure. Here, the consultant has asked for a scan to be ordered urgently and the form has been incorrectly filled out. The FY2 has dismissed you and it is now up to you to make sure the scan goes through. Calling the consultant to explain the situation (**A**), is the best option as they will be able to tell you what the scan is for. Asking the radiologist to call the consultant (**E**), is the next best idea as the FY2 (**D**) is clearly either busy or not bothered. It is not the best course of action as you have not taken steps to resolve the action yourself. **B** is generic advice and the other doctor has no part in this so will not be able to help and **C** contradicts guidelines on ordering investigations.

6. Answer:	BCDAE This question assesses the issues you might encounter around patient confidentiality and ethical issues at the end of life. Option **B** is most appropriate as there is an element of emotional/family conflict leading to this clinical scenario and encouraging the patient to speak to his family does not break confidentiality. Option **(C)** is also reasonable as his mental health could well have declined in 2 years with a progressive condition, however it would not necessarily help to resolve any family issues directly. Option **(D)** could only be considered if an updated liaison psychiatry assessment documented this. Option (**A**) and (E) involve breaching confidentiality, but **(A)** to a lesser degree than (**E**) which is the least appropriate option in this scenario.

7. Answer:	CEDBA This question addresses issues of patient capacity and autonomy. It is important to have a broad discussion when a patient is refusing their medication, to cover their concerns and understanding of the condition. Option **C** is the most appropriate, as it allows Boris to have his concerns addressed and explains the potential risks of untreated hypertension. Option **E** is less forceful but could be a potential compromise solution if the patient was adamant about homeopathy and gives a sensible timescale to revisit the GP and arrange follow-up care. Referring the patient back to GP **(D)** is vague and has no real element of addressing the patient's concerns directly, although the GP is likely to do this. **B** is correct, in that if Boris has capacity, he can refuse treatment but it is important to always attempt to engage the patient in their own care and ensure they understand their condition. Option **A,** while tempting, will negatively impact the doctor patient relationship and make Boris less likely to engage with medication in the future.

8. Answer:	ECDAB This is assessing your professionalism and ability to maintain good relationships. The most important action to take is to speak to your consultant **(E)** followed by contacting your medical defence union for advice **(C).** There is no particular need to contact the GMC **(D)** at this stage but it is less likely to cause additional damage than the other remaining options. Asking for witness evidence **(A)** could reflect badly on you, as you may be seen as interfering with the investigation into the complaint. By far the least appropriate option is to contact the relative directly **(B),** as this will escalate the situation further.

9. Answer:	BCAED This question assesses your reliability and commitment, as well as honesty and knowing your limits to be a safe doctor. The most important factor in this scenario is maintaining your own safety, and second to this comes the duty to patients. Honest communication with your team is the best way forward, and using public transport is the safest for you, so option **B** is most appropriate overall. Waiting to feel better is another option but may result in a lot of time being missed so **C** is less appealing. Calling in sick **(A)** would be partially appropriate however, if you are well enough to work, this could be potentially dishonest. It is a better answer than **E** which is a lie. The least appropriate option is **D** as this compromises your safety and the safety of others on the roads.

10. Answer:	DBACE This is a question concerning both patient and public safety. Epilepsy can make patients unsafe to drive and so there is a requirement to inform the DVLA. The most appropriate option is to tell the patient you must inform the DVLA but attempt to get their consent **(D).** If this cannot be achieved, you must still report their condition, making **B)**the next best option. It is an option to involve the GP in negotiations **(A)** but this may still fail and lead to you having to contact the DVLA without consent at a later date, increasing the risk to other drivers. Contacting the GP is however more likely to be successful than writing to the patient **(C),** however it is likely neither option will lead to success. The least appropriate option is to only report the patient to the DVLA with consent **(E)** as this leads to a delay.

11. Answer:	CADBE This is a test of confidentiality and dealing with other healthcare professionals. Being a doctor herself does not grant the FY1 special access to confidential information about patients who are not in her care. It would be most appropriate to explain that he is fine but that you cannot reveal more specific information as this is confidential **(C).** Explaining that you're unsure about the confidentiality rules so directing her to the consultant **(A)** would be the next best answer, as this means you are not breaching any rules. The remaining options all involve revealing confidential information so are not appropriate, but for this purpose you should rank them in the order that reveals the least information. So, the handover **(D)** would only contain information about his current status, telling her all the information about this admission **(B)** is more information than in the handover, and the least appropriate option is **E,** as this grants her access to his full medical history.

12. Answer:	ACBDE This question assesses commitment to patient care and the understanding that it ultimately trumps social commitments in this instance. The most appropriate action is **(A),** as this does not show signs of being a regular occurrence and it would be best for patient care to perform the handover in person. **(C)** is less appropriate but still ensures a face-to-face handover, where your colleague can flag up issues they are unsure of. **(B)** is less appropriate than C as it forgoes the face-to-face commitment of a handover, and your colleague may not be able to locate the list in an office that is not solely for your department. **(D)** is inappropriate as you are lying to a colleague who is likely already working hard on the busy shift, however it is still better than E as a handover will at least occur. **(E)** is very inappropriate as it shows poor teamwork and dangerously compromises patient care by omitting a handover altogether.

13. Answer:	DEABC This question assesses the ability to acknowledge a patient's concerns and worries as well as recognising your limits. The most appropriate action is **(D)** as you can alleviate some of her stress by giving her a plan of action, whilst not giving false promises or bypassing the necessity to get guidance from a superior. **(E)** also recognises your limits but will do less to alleviate her stress until the registrar arrives. **(A)** does address her concerns, but in an unhelpful way and does not explain how she will progress in terms of care and treatment. **(B)** addresses her concerns in an untruthful way and involves lying to a patient. **(C)** does not address her concerns and endangers the patient by ignoring her situation.

14. Answer:	BECDA This question assesses the ability to make professional decisions whilst not compromising working relationships. **(B)** is the most appropriate action as your consultant made the decision about the antibiotics, and avoids the pharmacist having to contact and explain the situation to another member of your team, as would occur in (**E**). After this, **(C)** would be the next most appropriate thing to do as it allows a professional to review the case and use their experience to perhaps understand complexities about this specific case you are not aware of. **(D)** ignores the fact that you are working as part of Dr Michaels' team and this team is who is directly responsible for the patients' care, thus endangering patient care. **(A)** does not address the problem and again can endanger patient care.

15. Answer:	CBAED This question assesses communication in the challenging situation of potentially breaking bad news but not having the required information. **(C)** is the most appropriate action as the senior colleague will have experience with his case and can discuss the diagnosis. **(B)** still addresses his concerns, but whilst you may have the test results, you will likely not have the knowledge to provide a thorough diagnosis and treatment options. **(A)** still addresses his concerns truthfully, but you neglect other patients and inconvenience another colleague, when you will likely have to get a senior colleague to have the discussion with Mr Crookes later. **(E)** is not appropriate as the diagnosis has not been confirmed, but **(D)** is the least appropriate as it involves lying to a patient and providing false hope when the likelihood is a recurrence.

16. Answer:	ABCED This question assesses patient care, confidentiality and patients' trust in the profession. Patient care is the priority that requires urgency in terms of correction. **(A)** alerts the patients more directly and gives a chance for you to apologise, and means inappropriate care is less likely to be given as the patient is aware of the mix up. **(B)** allows for patient care to be restored but doesn't give scope for an apology which is in order. Whilst **(C)** is good in that it seeks peer advice, it is better to speak to a more senior colleague in this case as patient care is at risk, especially as they have been discharged into the community. Both E and D are not appropriate and are unprofessional but **(D)** is the least appropriate of all options as it does not address the situation at all, i.e. allows no room for the GP to correct the mistake, and threatens patient care.

17. Answer:	ABCDE This question addresses aspects of patient confidentiality as well as knowing the appropriate way to approach a colleague. The most appropriate action is **(A)** as it will allow the post to be taken down immediately, and will allow you to have a conservation directly to explain why it was wrong to post. **(B)** also solves the problem, however it can be better to talk to them directly, seeing as this was the first occurrence. **(C)** still deals with the issue of lack of respect for patients, but escalates the issue far too much, especially as it is the first time this has happened. **(D)** is inappropriate as it does not solve the problem at hand and means patients may still be able to view the post in question. **(E)** is inappropriate as it does not solve the problem. It in fact suggest you agree with the post as 'likes' are publicly available to view and may encourage more of these posts.

18. Answer:	DBAEC This question looks at communication skills and how to communicate with team members professionally. In this instance, especially as this behaviour occurs in front of patients, concern and action is valid. The most appropriate option is **(D)** as Lucas might not even be aware of what he is doing, and a discussion could resolve the issue. **(B)** can be useful, as someone with experience may have experienced something similar before, but it does not address the issue in the way D does. **(A)** will not address the issue directly, but it does allow you to reflect and see what the issue is perhaps with both parties, and is a better option than E or C. **(E)** is inappropriate as it is unlikely after 2 weeks that anything will change, and it may have an effect on the patients' level of trust to see Lucas' behaviour. **(C)** is the least appropriate as it does not even attempt to solve an issue that may be simple, and doesn't allow you to develop any teamwork skills for such occasions as this.

19. Answer:	DBACE This question assesses issues of patient confidentiality and communication skills regarding this. The most appropriate action is **(D)** as you do not have consent to share this information and it is appropriate conduct as it does not involve lying to Mr Roach. The next option is **(B)** as it only shares information you have been given consent to share and allows you to have some time to ask Mrs Roach how she would like to proceed (and to indeed tell her about the results first). **(A)**is not ideal as it will likely stress out Mr Roach and place Mrs Roach in an immediately stressful situation, however it does not breach patient confidentiality. **(C)** is also evasive and may add stress to the situation, however again it does not break confidentiality. **(E)** is entirely unprofessional as, although it is truthful, it breaks confidentiality and Mrs Roach herself does not even know of the result yet.

20. Answer:	DBECA This question assesses your ability to recognise legitimate consent and mental capacity, especially in the case of elderly patients who may be unable to retain the information. The most appropriate option is **(D)** as it allows you to assess whether the patient does understand the operation and other options available. The next option is **(B)** which is less preferable to D as you can be such it is completed adequately if you have the discussion yourself. **(E)** is appropriate in the sense that the consultant has the ultimate responsibility, but it is unnecessary to go to him in the first instance and you should attempt to solve the issue before this step. **(C)** is inappropriate without attempting to solve the issue as the operation is likely in his best interest. **(A)** is the least appropriate action as no attempt has been made to solve the problem and you could be cancelling an operation important to his health.

21. Answer:	CDABE In this question it is important to understand how concerned the parents would be about their child's condition and not to take personal offence at the reaction. The most appropriate action to begin with is **(C)** to try and de-escalate the situation away from other patients and apologise - it is understandable how worried they are. **(D)** is less helpful than C as there is no apology but might help them understand the situation by giving the rationale. **(A)** may reduce the anger towards you but does not provide any apology or explanation. Although it is her right to complain, **(B)** is not as appropriate because she may be satisfied once an explanation and apology is given. **(E)** is the least appropriate thing to do as it does nothing towards calming the mother's anger, and unfairly places blame on the radiology department.

22. Answer:	CBDAE This question assesses your ability to recognise legitimate consent and mental capacity, especially in the case of elderly patients who may be unable to retain the information. The most appropriate option is **(D)** as it allows you to assess whether the patient does understand the operation and other options available. The next option is **(B)** which is less preferable to D as you can be such it is completed adequately if you have the discussion yourself. **(E)** is appropriate in the sense that the consultant has the ultimate responsibility, but it is unnecessary to go to him in the first instance and you should attempt to solve the issue before this step. **(C)** is inappropriate without attempting to solve the issue as the operation is likely in his best interest. **(A)** is the least appropriate action as no attempt has been made to solve the problem and you could be cancelling an operation important to his health.

23. Answer:	EDCBA This question assesses your ability to comfort a patient and reassure them. **(E)** is the most appropriate action as you can specifically comfort this patient and directly address his concerns to reduce his stress. **(D)** still allows you to directly reassure him but doesn't allow the discussion that E does, so may be less comforting. **(C)** will still address the issue but it is unnecessary to ask the nurse to do so as you are equipped to handle this, and you cannot be sure how long it will take for them to see him. **(B)** is not acceptable as you are not directly addressing the patient's concerns. **(A)** is the least appropriate as you could easily improve the patient care with a simple conversation so neglecting this is unprofessional.

24. Answer:	BADEC This question assesses how to communicate effectively with colleagues in a multi-disciplinary team. The most appropriate answer is **(B)** as it allows you to attend the round and if the nurse needs the task urgently completed, she can organise someone else to do it. **(A)** does not compromise patient care, but does mean you may miss out on information about other patients (however, you could catch up with notes) so it is less ideal. **(D)** demonstrates less effective communication, as you do not explain the situation and could lead to conflict. **(E)** shows unprofessional communication, especially in a busy ward, however it does not risk patient care in the way C does. **(C)** is the least appropriate as it involves lying to a colleague and if the job was urgent you may be placing the patient at risk by pretending it was done.

25. Answer:	DBACE This question assesses your response to an acutely sick patient. The best way to enhance patient safety is to rapidly perform an ABCDE assessment and start any basic treatment you think is appropriate. After you have done this, you can call for senior help. The best response is **(D)**, as you are assessing the patient immediately with another doctor- it's good to assess acutely sick patients with someone else, especially if you are not very experienced. **(B)** is also appropriate, although you are going on your own. **(A)** introduces a delay, which could have severe implications on the patient. **(C)** is clearly inappropriate and could lead to severe patient harm or even death. However, **(E)** is the worst option, as you are leaving the ward for an extended period of time when there is an acutely sick patient under your care.

26. Answer:	ADF This is a child safeguarding issue and should be handled appropriately and with care. You must wake the mother to ask her about the bruises (**A**) – she may provide you with a reasonable explanation for them that has been documented before in the notes (**D**). You must also carry out a full assessment (**F**) of the child to determine whether he has any serious injuries or hidden injuries.

27. Answer:	BCH This question assesses your communication skills. You must report the incident to the ward sister so appropriate disciplinary action can be taken (**B**). The incident must also be dealt with immediately as the nurses are demonstrating a serious lack of professionalism and are harming the reputation of the hospital (**C**). You must also reassure the other customers as they are clearly uncomfortable with the behaviour displayed by the nurses (**H**).

28. Answer:	EBC If you decide to go home that day, it is worth informing your team that you are going home, and which patients haven't been seen, so they can cover for you (**C**). Getting a locum to cover for you is a good idea because they can support the team while you are off sick. It demonstrates that you are thinking about the team and have a good team working skills (**B**). Remember you need to look after your own health, you may be dehydrated so drink some water(**E**),

29. Answer:	DBC This question assesses your communication skills. Asking her to rest her hip isn't enough (**D**), you need to explain to her why she should be resting as it's clear she may not have understood or listened to the initial instructions (**B**). Using clear and concise language is important here. You should also let her know when it's appropriate for her to walk around and when it isn't, and why (**C**).

30. Answer:	HAE You need to de-escalate the situation as you are alone, and Michael is being aggressive. You need to reassure him that you are there to help (**H**). Telling the truth is important here as Michael clearly needs support for what could be substance misuse. You need to help him access the right care and ensure that he is not compromising patient safety (**A**). Before reporting him, you need to get his side of the story so that he is willing to access care and ascertain if and why he is using drugs (**E**).

31. Answer:	CDE While the neighbours likely know the patient well there is no evidence that you can break patient confidentiality and discuss his care with them. They may be able to help you contact his son (E) who is more likely to be aware of powers of attorney. You must also check if there any documents that cite any pre-arranged agreements regarding Mr Hammon's care such as a DNAR for example (**C and D**).

32. Answer:	AHE You must inform the patient that there will be a student present during the consultation (**A**) and gain their consent for this (**H**). The patient must be able to make an informed decision so introducing the student is also appropriate so that the patient knows who the student is and why they are there (**E**).

33. Answer:	ADF The student is competent and can confidently talk you through the procedure. Thus, there should be no issue about letting her do the procedure. It is important that you explain to the patient that the medical student is going to catheterise him and gain his consent (**A** and **F**). You must also observe the student as she catheterises the patient to ensure that no mistakes are made (D).

34. Answer:	ABE You should support your colleagues and try to help them resolve issues as much as you are able. Reassuring him and providing comfort is not only a nice thing to do, but it also demonstrates good team working skills (**A**). Offering to speak to the consultant to get him extra support is appropriate, as the consultant may wish to re-delegate tasks to support the registrar or speak to him about the issue (**B**). A few days off may give the registrar some time to sort things out at home or find support networks that he can access should he wish to (**E**).

35. Answer:	DEC Discussing what happened with your consultant can get you valuable advice on what to do if this situation happens again (**D**). Reflecting on this episode and making a conscious effort to rectify it, can help you avoid incidents like this (**C** and **E**).

36. Answer:	BCD This question tests your ability to deal with hospital complaints and your patient-assurance skills. It is important that you find out the truth so you can tell the patient whether the reports are true or false **(C).** Furthermore, assuring the patient that she will be cared for well at the hospital is very appropriate, because that is as far as your knowledge goes **(B).** Similarly, asking Melissa how she feels would allow her to feel like she has been listened to, **(D),** although it does not solve the immediate problem of Melissa wanting to be moved to another hospital.

37. Answer:	BFC Although it may seem uncomfortable to automatically assume that she is lying, it may be necessary to ask her to tell the truth considering the severity of domestic abuse **(B).** To make it easier to do so, it may be important to have a conversation with her and ask if there is anyone at home who she is afraid of; opening up in this way can get her closer to revealing the truth behind her bruises **(C).** Similarly, it is vital to ensure that there is not anyone else at home who could be at risk from such abuse, especially children **(F)**. But it is important to consult with the patient first before making assumptions and calling social services or the police, which could break the trust the patient has on you.

38. Answer:	CGF This question tests your ability to deal with patients who you may have close relations with, and to speak the truth about the hospital care without jeopardising the reputation of your colleagues, or the confidence of your patient. It is often harder to lie to your closer relatives about the quality of their hospital care, but it is important to note that Mr. Sanders punctuality should not affect the quality of his work. You should tell the patient this, regardless of your relationship with the patient **(C & F).** At the same, you should reassure her that there will be no impact on her treatment **(G).**

39. Answer:	DHG It is important to first calm the patient down **(D).** It is important to value what she is saying and try to find a second opinion **(H),** On another note, it is also vital to understand what the nature of the patient's fears are, since knowing this may help to alleviate some of the concern she has about the operation **(G).**

40. Answer:	ACF This question tests your ability to ensure patient safety is prioritised at all times, which poor patient notes can jeopardise. It is important to try and contact Kate immediately and inform her that her notes are illegible as she has a responsibility for good note keeping and handover (A)(C). It is also worth speaking to a senior doctor for advice (F)

41. Answer:	EHG The patient is clearly agitated, the first thing to do would be to calm them down and/or ask her why she is experiencing discomfort with the nurse **(E).** The immediate problem right now is that the patient is not taking her tablets since she does not know why she needs them; therefore, the importance of her medication must be explained to her so that she feels more in control of her treatment **(H).** It may also be important to reassure the patient of the competence of the nurse, so that she is not blinded by any suspected prejudice **(G).**

42. Answer:	HGF If other staff members or patients catch Lila sleeping in the supply cupboard, it could reflect poorly on the profession and the hospital. Therefore, it is not appropriate to allow her to continue sleeping there. The most appropriate action is to remind Lila that she might be an obstacle for staff members who will want to get something from the cupboard on this busy night, **(H),** but this should be done in a polite and gently manner, since she is clearly going through a difficult time. Since you know that her financial situation is not great, he could offer her money to get a room at a local hotel **(F).** Alternatively, since it is just one night, it would be appropriate to allow Lila to sleep at his flat; this would ensure that she does not continue finding inappropriate places to sleep **(G).**

43. Answer:	DFE This question tests your ability to deal with conflict and difficult, and possibly prejudiced, patients. Since the patient is clearly agitated, the first thing to do would be to calm them down **(D).** The immediate problem right now is that the patient does not know how many people are before her in the queue, so that should also be told to her **(F).** Since she might be making others uncomfortable, it also may be wise to ask her if she would like to discuss her thoughts in privately, since that might help her to calm down whilst taking her away from the rest of the patients temporarily **(E).**

44. Answer:	FGC This question tests your ability to prioritise patient safety at all times. It also examines whether you will be able to maintain the reputation of yourself, your colleagues and the hospital, such that patient confidence and trust in the profession are not undermined. Although it is very likely that he could be drunk, it is important that you do not just confront Kieran and make assumptions. The most appropriate thing to do is to first ask him if he is okay and why he seems the way he is **(F).** To allow Kieran to continue to see the patient in his current state would put the patient at severe risk, and so it is advisable that he goes home **(G).** It is important to advise Kieran and give him a chance to explain first before going to the consultant. Kieran should also be given the chance to tell the consultant himself first **(C).**

45. Answer:	CEG This question tests your ability to deal with pressure and ensure the safety of yourself, your colleagues and the other patients. Although violence in a hospital environment is not acceptable, it is important to remember that this patient is suffering from delirium tremens, in which the patient is confused and agitated, so he would not actually understand that what he is doing is morally wrong. It would be appropriate to call security to ensure that another staff or patient are not hurt **(C).** It is important to try and calm the patient down and reduce the amount of emotion and tension **(E).** It is also important to ensure the safety of the other staff and check if any harm has been done to them **(G).**

46. Answer:	DEG This question tests ability to resolve conflict with friends and colleagues. You know that Jennifer should not be taking supplies and you should tell her this (D) and that you will raise with a senior if she doesn't stop (G). Jennifer's reasoning is commendable however there are more appropriate ways of helping the hospital in Zimbabwe and thus she should be signposted to HR (E)

47. Answer:	BCE You have to be honest with the patient and explain the situation and that you cannot discharge her (B). It is worth exploring Wanda's concerns and discussing this with her (C). It would be appropriate to try and contact the consultant as they may be able to give an indication of when they will return (E)

48. Answer:	ABE Your emotional wellbeing is important and thus you should be able to leave to see your grandmother (A). However this has to be done safely. (B) and (E) represents a safe handover of responsibilities before leaving.

49. Answer:	CGH This question tests your ability to handle an acute situation. The patient's health takes priority over discharge planning. A full neurological examination is required (G) accompanied by a MRI request (G) and informing the consultant (C)

50. Answer:	DEG The patient may still be at risk if there is hot liquid on the table and is unlikely to be able to clean it up himself. You should do this for him (D) and then make sure the nurse knows to help him with his coffee (E). It may be difficult to raise issues with colleagues however it would be worth feeding this problem back to the other doctor as they may not have realised what they had done (G)

CLINICAL PROBLEM SOLVING ANSWER KEY

1. E
2. B
3. D
4. C
5. A
6. F
7. E
8. H
9. C
10. A
11. E
12. B
13. C
14. E
15. G
16. A
17. C
18. D
19. B
20. D
21. C
22. D
23. B
24. A
25. A
26. B
27. B
28. A
29. C
30. G
31. G
32. D
33. A
34. D
35. A
36. C
37. A
38. G
39. B
40. F
41. C
42. C
43. B
44. C
45. A
46. C
47. C
48. B
49. C
50. C
51. E
52. A
53. C
54. D
55. E
56. E
57. D
58. A
59. F
60. C
61. D
62. B
63. A
64. E
65. A
66. D
67. G
68. H
69. E
70. C
71. C
72. D
73. C
74. A
75. D
76. E
77. B
78. D
79. D
80. B
81. D
82. E
83. C
84. A
85. H
86. B
87. C
88. D
89. D
90. B
91. D
92. C
93. B
94. E
95. A
96. C
97. D

APPLICATION SCORES

In order to decide applicant ranking, the MSRA scores from all the GP applicants are averaged around a mean score of 250 with a standard deviation of 40. There is also a minimum acceptable standard for each paper and if candidates do not meet this then their application is unsuccessful.

Applicants' scores and their national rank is then published on the Oriel platform and if successful then an offer will be made. The offers are based on national rank so will be the highest available offer once the rank of the applicant is reached. Once an offer has been received the applicant has 48 hours to decide whether to accept, reject or hold. Holding is only relevant if another specialty application has been made alongside GP and the applicant wants to wait to see if they receive an offer from this specialty before they consider accepting their GP offer. There is also the ability to opt-in to an automatic upgrade where the applicant will be moved to a higher preference offer if it were to become available e.g. through other applicants rejecting that offer or being upgraded themselves.

Once an offer is accepted then congratulations are in order and you can start to dream about the next stage in your career. The life of a GP trainee.

BEGINNING TRAINING

Starting specialty training can be a daunting experience however the GP pathway can be really rewarding. Most trainees have very little experience working as a GP before starting training, if any at all, and may have only two years of clinical experience out of medical school. Many foundation year placements are senior led, dominated by consultant or registrar ward rounds. In general practice it is usually only you and the patient in the consultation and thus you need to be able to lead the consultation and make decisions for their care. This is a skill that may not have been tested before.

Fortunately the GP training programme is called training for a reason. It is not expected when you start that you can consult and make decisions like a qualified GP. The goal is that the skills that you have demonstrated in the application process can be nurtured over the three years. This is a process that all GPs that you work with have had to go through and have succeeded in and you will be able to as well.

The programme is a mixture of posts in hospital and general practice and is assessed through a combination of Workplace Based Assessments (WPBA) and the MRCGP exam. The exam consists of the Applied Knowledge Test (AKT) and the Clinical Skills Assessment (CSA). Due to the Covid-19 pandemic the CSA has been replaced by the Recorded Consultation Assessment (RCA). At this time it is not clear if this will be a permanent change, whether the CSA will be introduced or whether a new hybrid examination will be produced. The MRCGP exam is taken in the later years of training and this guide will focus on the WPBAs and achieving a good start to training. With this you will be in a better position once the exams are due.

THE EPORTFOLIO

Always to draw a groan when mentioned, the ePortfolio is a necessary component of the training pathway and is the place where you have to demonstrate that you are achieving the competencies required. It is easy to bury one's head in the sand and put it to one side while concentrating on the more rewarding and interesting aspects of patient care. It is also much easier to complete if you work at it and take opportunities as you go along rather than rushing to get things signed off at the end of the year.

Most trainees will already have experience with portfolios in their careers, whether in foundation training or previous specialisation. The GP ePortfolio is taken especially seriously in assessing performance due to the relative remoteness of the training programme. An CT1 surgical trainee, for example, will be working consistently in surgical jobs with seniors who are familiar with their training programme and what it takes to become a surgeon. An ST1 GP trainee may spend up to 8 months of the year in hospital posts with seniors who are less likely to understand what it takes to be a GP. Their feedback is important however a lot more emphasis is put on the trainee to demonstrate they are meeting the competencies required for a GP. Unfortunately you could be a great doctor on an endocrine ward but if you are missing a competency at the annual review you are likely to be marked as making insufficient progress in training.

The platform for the ePortfolio is called Fourteen Fish (the reason for this name is indeterminate). It is surprisingly clear, intuitive and easy to use. It gives good representation of the capabilities achieved and your progress towards your next review and further ahead to completion of training.

Capability areas

There are thirteen capability areas that trainees are expected to link evidence to at each biannual review.

1. Fitness to practice
2. Maintaining an Ethical Approach
3. Communication and consultation skills
4. Data gathering and interpretation
5. Clinical examination and procedural skills
6. Making a diagnosis/ decisions
7. Clinical management
8. Managing medical complexity
9. Working with colleagues and in teams
10. Maintaining performance, learning and teaching
11. Organisation, management and leadership
12. Practising holistically, promoting health and safeguarding
13. Community orientation

This may seem like a lot but with a focussed and pragmatic approach towards the portfolio it is very achievable. Remember that if it is not evidenced in the portfolio then you have not demonstrated that capability.

Clinical experience groups

To demonstrate that you are receiving a satisfactorily broad training, there are 9 Clinical Experience Groups that you are expected to show coverage in when completing Workplace Based Assessments and Learning Logs.

- Infants, children and young people (under the age of 19)
- Gender, reproductive and sexual health (including women's, men's, LGBTQ+, gynaecology and breast)
- People with long term conditions including cancer, multi-morbidity and disability
- Older adults including frailty and/or people at end of life

- Mental health (including addiction, alcohol and substance misuse)
- Urgent and unscheduled care
- People with health disadvantage and vulnerabilities (including veterans, mental capacity difficulties, safeguarding and those with communication difficulties/ disability)
- Population health and health promotion (including people with non-acute and/or non-chronic health problems)
- Clinical problems not linked to a specific clinical experience group

Coverage of these areas is easier to attain than the capability areas. It is good to get a balance between the areas however some may be receive more coverage at times e.g. while on a Paediatrics placement it is likely there will be more relating to Infants, children and young people. Some coverage of all areas is expected at review so it is good to monitor for any gaps.

WORKPLACE BASED ASSESSMENTS (WBPAS)

This is the way that progress is continually assessed throughout the training programme and are times when someone else is completing this assessment. Some examples of capability areas that these assessments are good for covering have been given however any assessment has the potential to cover any capability area.

Case Based Discussion (CbD)

This is usually completed through a conversation with a senior doctor about a case that you have independently managed. It is good to pick a case that is interesting and gives opportunity to demonstrate capabilities such as managing medical complexity and maintaining an ethical approach.

- Managing medical complexity
- Maintaining an ethical approach
- Clinical management

These need to be completed in hospital posts. The doctor completing the assessment has to be ST4 or above. This can be frustrating when working with ST3 registrars in hospital posts who are keen to help you and are likely to be able to complete assessments for the trainees in their specialty.

Mini Clinical Evaluation Tool (MiniCEX)

In this assessment a patient interaction is observed and assessed while in a hospital post. The assessor then has the opportunity to give feedback on performance. Try and demonstrate capability in data gathering and interpretation, clinical examination and making a diagnosis.

Again, the doctors completing this must be ST4 or above.

- Data gathering and interpretation
- Clinical examination and procedural skills
- Making a diagnosis/ decisions
- Clinical management

Consultation Observation Tool (COT)

This is the equivalent of a MiniCEX while in a GP placement. As it is likely that the assessor will be a clinical supervisor with knowledge of the programme there is more opportunity for them to assess and give feedback. Audio-COTs can also be completed which are an assessment of your consultation over telephone. As well as demonstrating the capabilities mentioned when completing the MiniCEX, this can be a good opportunity to show communication and consultation skills.

- Data gathering and interpretation
- Clinical examination and procedural skills
- Making a diagnosis/ decisions
- Communication and consultation skills
- Clinical management

Clinical Examination and Procedural Skills (CEPS)

During training there are five intimate examinations that have to be observed and assessed as competent in order to complete training. These are:

- Breast examination
- Rectal examination
- Prostate examination
- Male genital examination
- Female genital examination

Although you have the three years to complete these examinations it is best to think about them early on. A bit of forward planning is required to find a patient who requires the relevant examination and then to get someone to observe. For example, it is unlikely that a GP will be able to take time out of the middle of a busy clinic to observe but may be more happy if planned ahead at the start or end of clinic.

These examinations can be completed in GP and hospital posts and the assessment can be done by a specialist nurse who has been specifically trained in the examination.

You can also complete a CEPS for other examinations and procedures that you complete and want to demonstrate competence in. This can help to show evidence of progress even if the procedure may not be immediately relevant to general practice. For example, you may learn and be observed performing a lumbar puncture in a hospital post. Although it is unlikely that you will do this during a clinic it still demonstrates evidence in your portfolio of clinical examination and procedural skills.

Multisource Feedback (MSF)

This is anonymised feedback that is given by other clinicians, healthcare professionals and administration staff that you work with on a day-to-day basis. It focusses on clinical performance and professional behaviour. You need to get at least 10 responses and 5 of them have to be clinicians. Once completed your educational supervisor will review the feedback and release the comments to yourself. There will also be a score that compares your feedback against other trainees.

It is usually preferable to complete this while in your GP placement as it is likely that you will be working with a more consistent team. It gives you an opportunity to demonstrate fitness to practice, working with colleagues and in teams and maintaining performance which can be difficult capabilities to achieve sufficient evidence.

Unless there are significant issues in the feedback, and these should be addressed by your educational supervisor, it is not worth getting too concerned by the MSF results but take on board any constructive criticism. It is a very blunt indicator of progress throughout the training programme and the score given can easily be influenced by few responses. It is best to reflect on the feedback and try to improve where necessary.

- Maintaining performance, learning and teaching
- Fitness to practice

Learning event analysis (LEA)

Being able to analyse both what went well and what could be improved is important for a GP. This assessment is a written reflection on an event or case that is likely to generate learning and will have a positive change to your, or your team's, practice going forward. This case is likely to fall beneath the GMC threshold for a Significant Event where there needs to be potential or actual serious harm to a patient.

It is better to choose an event that you are personally involved in as this will likely lead to a better quality reflection. Often the causes of events are multifactorial and thus it is important to consider the bigger picture.

Example:

Title: Interaction of clopidogrel and omeprazole

<u>What happened, including your role?</u>

I reviewed a 65 year old male patient in the GP surgery. He presented with epigastric pain which worsened after eating. From the history and examination there were no red flags and I treated him for dyspepsia with a one month course 20mg omeprazole daily and booked him for a follow up appointment to assess his symptoms. One week later I was contacted by the practice pharmacist who informed me that she had asked the patient to stop taking the omeprazole as he was also taking clopidogrel due to a myocardial infarction 6 months ago and there is an interaction between these medications, potentially reducing the effectiveness of the clopidogrel. He had been changed to lansoprazole which is safer.

Why did it happen?

I had not come across this interaction before in my clinical practice and therefore when prescribing I did not consider whether there was an interaction. It was a busy morning and I did not check the patient's current medication for potential interactions. Often when prescribing electronically there is a pop-up when there is a drug interaction and this did not occur.

What was done well?

I think that prescribing a proton pump inhibitor in this situation was an appropriate management plan. It was good that the pharmacist was able to recognise the prescription error and advised the patient to stop taking. This acted as a safety net for the error. Fortunately there was no patient harm from this event and the patient was very understanding.

What could be done differently?

I feel that I need to revise my knowledge of common drug interactions to reduce the chances of this happening again. I need to make sure that I always check for potential interactions when prescribing. I need to recognise that even if the clinic is busy it is still important to take my time and be thorough when prescribing, especially at my stage of training as I do not have much clinical experience.

Who was involved in the discussion of this event?

After the pharmacist told me about the interaction and my prescribing error, I discussed the event with my clinical supervisor. We agreed that I would present the event at the next practice meeting. This was attended by the practice manager, practice nurses and other GPs working at the practice.

What have you and the team learnt?

When I presented the event at the practice meeting I was surprised to find out that some of the other GPs were not aware of the interaction. They were grateful that I highlighted this issue and we all felt that this was an event everyone could learn from.

What changes have you or the organisation made?

Following the practice meeting an email was sent to all the clinicians reminding them of the interaction. The practice manager is going to make sure that an alert pops up on the electronic prescribing system if omeprazole is attempted to be prescribed for patients on clopidogrel. An audit has been carried out to make sure that there are not any patients on regular prescriptions of both the medications.

- Fitness to practice
- Maintaining performance, learning and teaching
- Organisation, management and leadership
- Practising holistically, promoting health and safeguarding

Quality Improvement Project (QIP)

The training programme is keen on developing doctors that can identify ways of improving the system that they work in, especially if this impacts on patient safety. There used to be more emphasis on audit completion however now a QIP is seen as more achievable in a four month placement. QIPs and audits are slightly different and it is useful to understand the difference between the models, especially if you have previously completed audit work.

The framework for QIPs is based on the Model for Improvement. This initially asks three questions of 'What are we trying to accomplish?' 'How will we know that a change is an improvement?' 'What change can we make that will result in an improvement?'. To enact this change, a cycle of Plan, Do, Study, Act is undertaken. This model is deemed to be quicker and less onerous than a traditional audit cycle.

The QIP can take place in primary or secondary care. It is usually easier to complete in primary care due to more computer-based record keeping and the RCGP recommends this. The choice of what QIP to undertake is a personal preference and it is advantageous if it can be linked to a frustration or learning need that you have identified. Your supervisor should be able to advice you on picking a suitable project.

Example of QIP project plan

Review of concordance with local guidelines in management of urinary tract infection in the over 65s in a GP practice

<u>What are we trying to accomplish? (Project aims)</u>
All prescriptions for urinary tract infections in over 65s at the practice to meet local guidelines

<u>How will we know that a change is an improvement? (Establishing measures)</u>
A retrospective search will be performed on the computer system for urinary tract infection diagnoses in patients over 65 in the practice over the previous month. The prescriptions will be compared with local guidelines. The percentage of prescriptions meeting local guidelines will be evaluated. An increase in this percentage following the change would indicate an improvement.

<u>What changes can we make that will result in improvement? (Selecting changes)</u>
The guidelines have recently changed and some clinicians may not be aware of this. Therefore education of the local guidelines may result in improvement.

Testing changes
Plan – Posters will be developed displaying the local guidelines
Do – The posters will be placed in every clinical room
Study – Another search will be completed evaluating the prescriptions in the month following the implementation of the posters
Act – The results will be discussed with the team at the practice meeting and further changes can be planned if necessary.

- Maintaining performance, learning and teaching
- Organisation, management and leadership
- Working with colleagues and in teams

Clinical supervisor report

At the end of every rotation your clinical supervisor needs to complete a report on your progress and this gives them an opportunity to highlight any concerns. It is a form that has sections on relationship (with patients and colleagues), diagnostics, management and professionalism. This is not something that supervisors, especially those in hospital, always remember to complete and therefore it is good to request a meeting to discuss a couple of weeks before the end of your placement. It can become difficult to chase supervisors for this after you have moved on from a placement as you are no longer in the department and they have a new cohort of trainees to supervise. It must be completed to progress with training.

Other WBPAs – these do not need to be completed in ST1 but are worth understanding while training

Leadership activity (ST3) –. Trainees propose their own activity that demonstrates leadership ability e.g. chairing a meeting. This then followed up with a reflective piece in the portfolio and an MSF.

Prescribing assessment (ST3) – 50 retrospective prescriptions are reviewed by the trainee and any prescribing errors are considered. The GP trainer then reviews 20 of these prescriptions and the findings are discussed.

Care Assessment Tool (5 in ST3) – These cover case based discussions in primary care as well other activities such as the prescribing assessment follow up, random case reviews or referral reviews

Patient satisfaction questionnaire (PSQ) (ST3) – A 9 part questionnaire for patients to complete after a consultation. At least 34 responses are required. A score is produced which can be compared to a peer average. Your educational supervisor will then release the results and you can discuss at a meeting.

General tips

- The doctor signing off a WBPA has to be ST4 or above. Be aware of this when working with junior registrars in hospital
- Everyone is always busy and therefore signing off your WBPA is often low on their to do list or they forget. Remember that you need these for your progression and career so don't be afraid to chase people up to get the sign off. People won't be offended and many will have been in your position themselves.
- Don't leave getting the WBPAs to be completed until the last minute. If you fail to get enough it will be noticed on review.
- Space out the WBPAs throughout the year. It will be apparent if it is all done in one placement.
- When completing the multi-source feedback, try and ask as many people as possible. Many people forget to fill in the feedback and, as it is anonymised, it can be difficult to chase people.
- Try and identify a QIP in the first couple of months of the GP placement, this gives ample time to complete the whole project.

LEARNING LOGS

These logs are your reflections on your practice. They give an opportunity to show evidence of the capability areas as well as being self-aware and honest about your progress.

Clinical case reviews

These form the core of the learning log part of the ePortfolio. 36 have to be completed each year. It is a good idea to keep completing these as you go. You need to complete approximately one every 10 days so it is easy to get behind. By completing them close to the time of seeing the case you will have a better memory of the case and this will improve the quality of your reflection. The clinical case reviews can be about anything patient based. It can be a patient interaction but it could also be a discussion with a relative or another member of the multidisciplinary team.

The logs have to be reflective and it is a better to talk about your feelings with regards to the case rather than just focussing on the medicine. You are able to provide evidence for 3 capabilities with every log so it is good to regularly review whether there are any gaps in your evidence and write a log to demonstrate evidence in that capability. Some areas, like community orientation, can be more difficult to provide evidence for so it is good to always be on the look out for relevant cases to review.

Example logs:

Title:
A palliative patient with metastatic lung cancer

Date:
08/03/2021

Setting:
Home visit

Brief description:
I went on a home visit to review an 80 year old gentleman who has been just discharged from hospital following a new diagnosis of metastatic lung cancer.

Clinical experience groups:
People with long term conditions including cancer, multi-morbidity and disability
Older adults including frailty and/or people at end of life

Example of a poor log entry:

Capability: Clinical management

Justification:
As this patient is palliative I needed to sort out their RESPECT form and anticipatory medications. I visited the patient's home and we discussed DNAR and completed the form. The anticipatory medications I prescribed were morphine, midazolam, levomepromazine and hyoscine butylbromide. I also stopped some of his medications that he does not need. I made sure he was on the practice palliative care register. I called the palliative care nursing team and they will review.

Reflection: What will I maintain, improve or stop?
I have made a note of the anticipatory medications so I won't forget them

Learning needs identified from this event:
Learn about palliative care

Example of a good log entry:

Capability: Communication and consultation skills

Justification:
I always find discussing end of life with patients difficult but this is improving with practice. I sat down with the patient and his wife and, after checking their understanding, discussed his prognosis. We spoke about what palliative and resuscitation means. The patient said he was a bit confused when it was discussed in hospital but feels it is clearer now and understands why resuscitation would not be appropriate. This made me feel like I had communicated effectively.

Capability: Clinical management

Justification:
During a palliative care review it is important to look at the patient's regular medications. I felt that it was appropriate to stop his statin and his antihypertensives at this point as they are for reducing long-term risk and this will reduce polypharmacy. He should still take his inhalers as it offers symptomatic relief however I can see this may become difficult as he gets frailer. It is uncertain what the patient's prognosis is. He does not require any anticipatory medication at this time but I have prescribed in case the situation changes.

Capability: Working with colleagues and in teams

Justification:
GP practices cannot offer all the services that a palliative patient requires. I felt that it was important to liaise with the palliative nursing team directly so that a team-based approach could be taken. They will be able to organise a syringe driver if required and can review the patient overnight and at weekends when the practice is closed. I also made sure the patient was on the practice palliative register as this communicates to my colleagues at the practice that palliative care plans have been made.

Reflection: What will I maintain, improve or stop?
This consultation went well but I think I will have more difficult conversations about dying in the future. I want to continue to improve the fluency with which I discuss these topics with patients

Learning needs identified from this event:
I feel that I need to understand more about palliative care – the local area prescribing committee have produced a guideline for end of life care and I intend to read this

TIPS FOR WRITING CLINICAL CASE REVIEWS

- Try to write about why you did something rather than just what you did
- Don't be afraid to write about how you felt even if this is not completely positive
- If something didn't go well – try and ask yourself how it can go better next time and write about this
- Keep an anonymised note of patients suitable to write case reviews about after the event as it is easy to forget about them
- You can link up to three capabilities to each case – try to maximise this to improve the body of evidence at review
- However, each capability needs to be justified so be wary of linking just for the sake of it. Look at the word descriptors for the capability to get inspiration for if it is appropriate.
- Remember this is a demonstration of your capabilities so try and write in a language that evidences this to those who read it.

Educational supervisor report (ESR)

At the end of every review period (usually six months if full time) there will be an educational supervisor report. This looks at how you are progressing with training and demonstrating improvement or competency in the capability areas. In order to prepare for the ESR you will need to complete an exercise called self-rating for each of the capability areas.

During self-rating you will need to give a rating of your performance in the capability area of either 'Needs further development', 'Competent' or 'Excellent'. This rating is in comparison to a fully qualified GP therefore in the first couple of years of training it is expected that you will mostly rate as 'Needs further development'.

Underneath the rating you need to provide evidence to support the rating. This is where good planning in completing WBPAs and Learning logs can pay off. You can link up to three entries as evidence and it is good to justify this. The word descriptors for the capability can be very useful here. You may want to discuss with your supervisor how they want you to display the evidence but an example may be:

Clinical management
Learning log 08/03/21 – 'During a palliative care review it is important to look at the patient's regular medications. I felt that it was appropriate to stop his statin and his antihypertensives at this point as they are for reducing long-term risk and this will reduce polypharmacy.' – This demonstrates capability in clinical management as I am confident in stopping medication where appropriate

You will also need to come up with at least 3 action plans for until the next review. These will be each linked to a capability area. It is best to try and vary the capability areas and to think about areas of weakness.

Your ESR preparation is reviewed by your educational supervisor and they will give their ratings and discuss with you about your action plan. Once they have completed their feedback and rating you will need to sign off the report to say you agree with the plan.

This table overleaf summarises the workplace based assessments for each year of training required (as of 2021)

WBPA	ST1	ST2	ST3
Mini-CEX/ COT	4	4	7
CBD/CAT	4	4	5
MSF	1	1	2 (1 leadership)
PSQ	0	0	1
CEPS	5 intimate required across the 3 years + others		
Learning logs (case reviews)	36	36	36
QIA	1	1	1
Learning event analysis	1	1	1
Prescribing assessment	0	0	1
Leadership activity	0	0	1
CSR	1 per post	1 per post	1 per post
ESR	2	2	2

WORKING AS A GP TRAINEE

By definition if you have elected to start the GP training programme your experience in General Practice will be limited. Some candidates may have done a rotation during their foundation years, some may not have any GP experience since medical school and some may have trained abroad in a very different healthcare system. The training programme caters to all.

GP practices are usually run as businesses that provide primary healthcare to an area on behalf of the NHS through a contract of services. They are often small but work with other local practices through a primary care network (PCN) and Clinical Commissioning group (CCG) to pool resources and present a strategy towards primary healthcare for the wider area. The average list size of a GP practice in England in 2019 was just over 9000 patients.

Compared to hospitals which cover very large populations and have hundreds or even thousands of staff members, an individual GP practice is on a much smaller scale. Due to this it is possible to have a close-knit workforce that knows the patients and the area well. It can use this as a strength to tailor its care towards the needs of its patients and the skills of its staff.

As a GP trainee your role is to learn, gain experience and grow as a clinician and your duties should reflect this. You are however still a part of that team and being able to train trainees is a source of pride for many GP practices. Patients are also often aware of GPs in training and are very accommodating of this, however remember you are still the face of the practice to the patient and your standards reflect on your host practice.

Although training practices are not homogenous they do have to be approved by a governing organisation e.g. Health Education England in England and meet certain standards. Although you will have an educational or clinical supervisor in the practice who will be a GP, you will receive training from the whole practice and it is important to understand the roles the other members of the practice play.

THE PRACTICE TEAM:

- Doctors
- Nurses
- Advanced Clinical Practioners (ACP)
- Healthcare assistants
- Pharmacists
- Physios
- Practice manager
- Reception staff
- Secretaries
- And more

As the role of a GP changes and becomes more managerial, the multidisciplinary team approach towards care becomes more important. Having a good relationship and understanding of the skills of the other members of the team will improve your skills as a GP. This is reflected by the GP programme in the need to regularly receive multi-source feedback.

SETTLING INTO TRAINING

The start of training can be daunting and frustrating. Even if you have a lot of experience working in hospital there is still likely to be a steep learning curve. It can feel isolating when it is just yourself and the patient in the consultation room and you don't know what is wrong with them. Apparently simple conditions can become minefields as you would have never encountered them before in this context. The recognition of normal and the patient's agenda becomes more important. Diagnostic uncertainty may not be able to be investigated to the depth or breadth that it can in secondary care. Don't worry!

It is understood that trainees are likely to feel this way and there are ways to try and improve the situation.

At the start of training the appointment time length is much longer than your fully trained colleagues. Often 30 minutes per patient is used at the start. This may seem like a long time compared to the infamous 10 minutes of a usual GP appointment however it allows for more considered history taking and a more lengthy examination which is required at this stage. Importantly it gives time to look things up after the consultation which is invaluable when the patient is still fresh in your mind.

As training progresses the appointment times will shorten and you will see more patients. There is no set timetable as to this occurring and is a discussion between yourself and the trainer. Don't compare yourself to other trainees at the practice or on the programme as it is not a good reflector of progress. Remember the goal is for safe patient care and gaining the skills required to be a GP not to just get patients through the door.

The opportunity to debrief your patients with a GP at the end of the session is a good way to get some feedback on your decision making. It is also a time where you can realise that there are many different clinical styles and by speaking to different GPs you can see which resonates with your way of working and may inspire your practice.

HOME VISITS

A full day working as a GP usually consists of a morning clinic and an afternoon clinic with time for admin and home visits in the middle. The number of home visits that a practice carries out depends on its population, for example there is likely to be few in a student area, and the practice policy. Although they can be unpopular due to the time cost of travelling to a patient's home, often it is the most vulnerable patients that require visits and thus it is a necessary part of the GP care.

Performing a consultation in a patient's home is a different experience to the GP surgery. Some of the crutches that we all use in day to day practice are gone. You don't have your computer to look up the patient's history, there is no examination couch so you have to improvise and you can't ask a colleague to pop in if you are unsure.

You also get an amazing view into how a patient lives. Patients often give a rose-tinted history of their social factors but on a home visit it is laid bare. You can see what environmental factors might be at play and build up a more holistic picture of the patient. It is also a tremendous privilege to be invited into someone's home.

Checklist before going on a home visit

1. Check your doctor's bag – make sure you have all the equipment that you need for the visit and that it works. Your ability to do a full assessment will be impaired if your oxygen saturation monitor is out of battery.
2. Look up the patient's history – it is good to take a print out a summary with the patient's medications, allergies and past medical history. It can be useful to check the past few consultations for the patient. Are they requiring frequent visits? Are there other teams involved in their care? Have advanced directives been put in place?
3. Make sure you have any contact numbers you will need – As patients requiring a home visit are more vulnerable, they are more likely to need admission to hospital. Put the contact details for local hospital admissions as well as the ambulance service into your phone. Also make sure you have your practice's number in case you need to get advice or more information.

URGENT AND UNSCHEDULED CARE

The demand for medical care never stops. Out of hours GP services help to carry the baton when practices are closed and can help to reduce the strain on emergency services. To reflect this, GP trainees need to demonstrate capabilities in managing urgent and unscheduled care. The best way to complete this may differ depending on geographical location and local services and the programme should give direction on this. There may be an out of hours service that you can work at and you may be able to demonstrate some competencies within your usual practice.

In essence patient care should be the same in hours and out. In practice this is not quite the case. From the patient's view they think that their problem is urgent enough to not be able to wait until their own GP practice is open and from the doctor's view there is more risk involved in out of hours care. Due to this a more cautious approach is often taken.

Often as a doctor we balance risk. A surgeon may weigh up the benefits of performing surgery against the risks of complications. An acute care physician may balance the effect of diuretics on a fluid overloaded patient against the potential harm to the kidneys. As a GP much of the risk comes from potential inaction. What if you have got the diagnosis wrong, reassured the patient and the patient goes home and comes to serious harm?

In an out of hours setting the potential for risk is higher for a few reasons. The patient has contacted thinking their problem is urgent which increases the likelihood that it actually is. Often the patient history known to the out of hours doctor is brief and they cannot access recent investigations such as blood tests. In usual practice you will get to know patients over time but there is no chance for this in urgent care. Defined follow up is also difficult to organise and can rely on letters to GP practices. Factors such as a more inconsistent team in out of hours and the possibility of the work environment being unfamiliar to the doctor also matter.

A GP needs to trust their judgement but also needs humility to understand that they are not perfect and even with all available evidence pointing one way the diagnosis may actually be something else. We make a differential diagnosis and weigh up what would be likely and what would be serious to miss. The vast majority of the time, common things are common and it is safe to reassure the patient that it is unlikely that their complaint is serious, at least from a medical point of view.

A good doctor has faith in their judgement but also uses safety netting to try to protect the patient and reduce the risk of serious harm. This involves informing the patient of the potential serious complications and what to do if these occur.

Example:

You have seen a patient with back pain in the out of hours clinic. It appears musculoskeletal in nature and there are no red flags. You have suggested anti-inflammatories and exercises and explained that you expect it to improve with your management plan.

This is a common scenario which often presents in general practice and this management plan is reasonable. In very rare cases patients can go on to develop cauda equina which is an emergency however there is nothing to indicate this would be the case at the time. Some patients, having been reassured after their assessment by a GP, may ignore worsening or new symptoms and suffer poor outcomes as a result. Safety netting helps educate the patient what to do if your diagnosis is wrong and the worst case scenario occurs. It needs to be specific and remember to document what you said to the patient in the notes.

'I think that your pain is in the muscles in your back and should improve with exercises and anti-inflammatory medication. In very rare cases back pain can be due to damage to the nerves at the bottom of the spine and this is an emergency. If you experience any symptoms of numbness in your groin, opening your bowels without knowing or if you are struggling to pass urine then head straight to the emergency department or call 999. I do not think this will happen but it is important for you to know what to do if it occurs.'

THE EXAMS

As you progress through GP training the prospect of exams starts to loom large. These competency exams are testing that the candidate is at the standard of a qualified GP and can demonstrate safe and independent practice. There is a knowledge exam, Applied Knowledge Test (AKT), and a consultation exam, Clinical Skills Assessment (CSA)/ Recorded consultation assessment (RCA).

As these are competency exams it is not expected that a trainee will have the skills required to pass until they have completed the majority of their training. The AKT can be taken in ST2 at the earliest and the CSA/RCA in ST3. When to take the exams is a personal preference and the important thing is completing them by the end of ST3. Bear in mind that the exams are eye wateringly expensive so retakes are best avoided.

Usually trainees complete the AKT first. This builds clinical knowledge that may then be tested in, but is not the focus of, the CSA/RCA. The AKT exam is similar in structure to the clinical problem solving paper of the MSRA but understandably is of a harder standard. It is a computer based assessment with multiple choice questions. Experience working in GP is useful but most of the preparation work is through revision.

For the CSA/RCA experience working as a GP is essential as it is testing your clinical skills. This can only be developed through seeing patients in general practice. The exam has an OSCE format and the candidate has to complete 13 consecutive ten minute consultations which simulate different GP scenarios.

The marks are split between data gathering, clinical management and interpersonal skills.

At the start of training it is good to be aware of the different exams but you do not need to think about them until ST2. The best preparation during the first year of training is through clinical experience and reflection on your consultation skills and what being a GP means to you.

AFTER TRAINING

Some trainees have a very strong idea from the start of what they are going to do once they complete training. Most however do not. General practice training is more open ended than other specialties where there is a long road to inevitable consultancy. A great advantage of being a GP is the ability to create a role that suits your interests and strengths. There is also greater flexibility to work less than full time to accommodate commitments outside of medicine.

GP roles tend to be defined by the number of sessions that the GP works in a week. The BMA defines a session as 4 hours and 10 minutes which includes the time to see the list of patients and admin related to this. A full time GP would work 9 sessions to complete a standard 37.5 hour week.

Commonly there are 3 different types of GP role:

Salaried GPs
These GPs are employed by a practice to complete a number of sessions per week. Working a salaried role means consistent work and you would get the employee benefits of annual leave and sick pay. As it tends to be a long term role there may be an expectation to take part in some of the wider administrative duties for the practice, for example audit work, but this would be defined in your contract.

Locum GPs

By working as a locum GP you would be contracted to perform a defined service to a practice for a set time. These tend to be short term, for example 2 sessions to cover a day sickness or a gap in a rota, but longer term locum roles exist if a GP is going to be away for a longer time such as on maternity leave. The advantages of working as a locum is the flexibility of which days that you work and pay tends to be higher. It can be challenging as you may be working in many different practices for short periods of time and thus cannot build a rapport with patients or the practice like those in a longer-term role. Work may be inconsistent and you would usually not receive the benefits of paid sick or holiday leave.

GP partners

The current model of primary care in the UK is for the NHS to contract individual GP practices to provide services for its local population. This means that one or a group of practices is a private business and this is owned by a sole or group of partners. GP partners have clinical responsibilities similar to a salaried GP in that they would complete a defined number of sessions per week. They would also have an expanded administrative role and may be involved in hiring staff, dealing with complaints and management decisions. Working as a GP partner can be well paid and is good if you want to be involved in the running of a practice. As you have the most responsibility in the practice it can mean long hours and increased stress.

Most GPs when completing their training take up either a salaried or locum position or even a combination of the two. When starting out as an independent practitioner it can be beneficial to have the consistency of a salaried job. Locums tend to have less support but the experience of working in multiple different practices can help to define what role you want in the future. While some trainees go straight into partnership after training, this is rare and it is considered normal to develop a few years of experience before taking on the extra responsibilities of this role.

OTHER GP ROLES

GPs with Extended Roles (GPwERs)

These used to be known as GPs with Special Interests (GPwSIs). These are GPs that undertake a role in another specialty in addition to their role as a general practitioner. These extended role takes place outside of the usual general practice setting and is likely to require further training and accreditation. Common examples would be Dermatology or gynaecology.

Medical education

Many GPs are interested in training future generations. The role of being a clinical or educational supervisor for the GP training programme can be easily combined with a core role as a GP. To become a GP trainer you will require at least 1 year experience working in a training practice, 2 if in a non-training practice, following completion of training. There are also opportunities to be involved in the training of medical students.

The true breadth of career opportunities available to GPs cannot be given justice on a page and it is always amazing to see what inspiring roles people have taken on. From academic research to management roles within the NHS, working in prisons or volunteering with the lifeboat service, the transferable skills developed as a General Practitioner means we can turn our hand at anything.

CONCLUSION

This book aims to give you the opportunity to get the most out of the start of your GP career. By achieving a high score at the MSRA and being successful in your application to your chosen programme you should be able to build a knowledge foundation that will help when improving your clinical skills during training. By engaging and keeping on top of the assessments in the portfolio during early training you will gain a lot more out of the scheme and it will hopefully make the Annual Review of Competency Progression (ARCP) much less stressful.

A successful training programme should mean growing in confidence as a clinician as well as passing the exams and assessments. It will mean being able to handle the wide range of problems that can come in through your consulting room door. Learning to be a GP is a lifelong endeavour and one sign of a good GP is a recognition of their own shortcomings. GP training will be a rewarding experience and the career path that you take onwards will be worthwhile.

WORK WITH UNIADMISSIONS

UniAdmissions is the UK's number one university admissions company, specialising in **supporting applications to Medical School and to Oxbridge**. Every year, *we* help thousands of applicants and schools across the UK. From free resources to these *Ultimate Guide Books* and from intensive courses to bespoke individual tuition, *UniAdmissions* boasts a team of **500 Expert Tutors** and a proven track record of producing great results.

UniAdmissions is always looking for enthusiastic tutors to help nurture tomorrow's talent. In addition to gaining valuable teaching and training skills, tutoring with us allows you to gain vital application points for your core medical or surgical training applications. All our medical tutors have the option of completing free teaching and training courses to help give their medical/surgical applications a much needed boost and stand out from the crowd.

In addition, you're guaranteed to earn more than £ 100 per day's work; to find out more visit: www.uniadmissions.co.uk/work-with-us

ABOUT US

We currently publish over 100 titles across a range of subject areas – covering specialised admissions tests, examination techniques, personal statement guides, plus everything else you need to improve your chances of getting on to competitive courses such as medicine and law, as well as into universities such as Oxford and Cambridge.

Outside of publishing we also operate a highly successful tuition division, called UniAdmissions. This company was founded in 2013 by Dr Rohan Agarwal and Dr David Salt, both Cambridge Medical graduates with several years of tutoring experience. Since then, every year, hundreds of applicants and schools work with us on our programmes. Through the programmes we offer, we deliver expert tuition, exclusive course places, online courses, best-selling textbooks and much more.

With a team of over 1,000 Oxbridge tutors and a proven track record, UniAdmissions have quickly become the UK's number one admissions company.

Visit and engage with us at:
Website (UniAdmissions): www.uniadmissions.co.uk
Facebook: www.facebook.com/uniadmissionsuk

YOUR FREE BOOK

Thanks for purchasing this Ultimate Book. Readers like you have the power to make or break a book –hopefully you found this one useful and informative. *The Oxbridge Medical Society* would love to hear about your experiences with this book. As thanks for your time we'll send you another ebook from our Ultimate Guide series absolutely FREE!

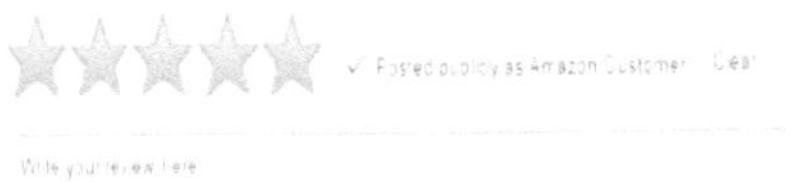

How to Redeem Your Free Ebook

1) Find the book you have on your Amazon purchase history or your email receipt to help find the book on Amazon.

2) On the product page at the Customer Reviews area, click 'Write a customer review'. Write your review and post it! Copy the review page or take a screen shot of the review you have left.

3) Head over to **https://www.uniadmissions.co.uk/oxbridge-free-book/** and select your chosen free ebook!

Your ebook will then be emailed to you – it's as simple as that!

Printed and bound by CPI Group (UK) Ltd, Croydon, CR0 4YY
02/11/2026
02243551-0002